Don't Let The Health Service Kill You

Jimmy Smyth

www.DontLetTheHealthServiceKillYou.com

Published in 2011 by
Jimmy Smyth
Newcastle
County Down

The author gratefully acknowledges the help given by Clive Scoular and Thomas Johnston in the creation of this book.

ISBN 978-0-9569314-0-5

for Gregory,
a kind and loving brother

About the author

Jimmy Smyth trained and worked in Downshire Hospital as a psychiatric nurse and in Epsom District Hospital as a general nurse. He then completed his social work training at the University of Ulster and later qualified as an approved social worker. Jimmy has worked in a number of areas within the Health Service for almost forty-years.

He is married with two daughters and a step-daughter and lives in the seaside town of Newcastle, County Down, having lived for most of his life in Kilkeel, County Down.

This is Jimmy's first book and he was motivated to write it as he believes that we need to become more aware of the importance of our health and we should play our part in helping to raise standards within health care.

His hobbies are reading, walking and holidaying in Spain.

Health is not a condition of matter, but of mind.

Mary Baker Eddy

dontletthehealthservicekillyou@gmail.com

Acknowledgements

My deepest gratitude to Kathryn and Amanda, for all the work they helped me with, for their advice and for putting up with me and listening to me, especially during the early hours of the morning.

Appreciation and thanks to my wife and family for their help, support, encouragement and patience.

To my mother, an incredible woman, who has inspired me throughout my life. Thanks mum.

Health is the greatest gift, contentment the greatest wealth, faithfulness the best relationship.

Buddha

Disclaimer

This book is designed to help you to gain a better understanding of the Health Service, to encourage you to change your thinking and attitude towards health care and to make your health your number one priority.

Every effort has been made to make this book as complete and as accurate as possible. However there may be mistakes, typographical and in content. Therefore this book should be used only as a general guide and not as an authority on health care.

The purpose of this book is to make you better informed about health care and to encourage you to become more proactive in pursuing your health care needs.

The author and publisher shall have neither liability nor responsibility to any person or entity with respect to any loss or damage caused or alleged to have been caused, directly or indirectly, by the information contained in this book.

Medicine sometimes snatches away health,

sometimes gives it.

Ovid

Contents

One:
Introduction

In the course of this book we will be looking in some detail at the medical services that are available to us and how we can get the most out of them. There is no doubt that we need to have a better understanding about how the NHS works.

We become a patient and we need to take steps to protect ourselves and our families from the mistakes that are made by doctors and hospitals. To protect ourselves against doctors' and hospitals' mistakes is as important as protecting ourselves against cancer, heart disease and other serious illnesses.

The NHS can do you a great deal of good but it can also do you a lot of harm. To increase your chances of getting the highest quality health care possible and to be knowledgeable about the range of services and treatment options that are available, you need to stop taking your health for granted. You need to become more proactive and become an equal partner with your doctor and hospital and actively pursue good preventive healthcare.

In life, getting enough money to have a great lifestyle and being successful is a priority for most people. We spend a large part of our lives studying, training, competing and whatever else it takes to have the money and lifestyle we yearn for.

Some people achieve their goals, but many people do not. In contrast, how much time do we spend focusing on leading healthy lives and maintaining our health? The truth for many of us is that we take our health for granted and do not even for a moment believe that we will ever be ill.

Even if illness knocks on our door, we are sure a trip to the doctor will put things right. Unfortunately it is not always that simple and even if we have been financially successful but neglected our health, then our money and success may suddenly become meaningless.

Regularly it is reported in the media of people dying as a result of 'Doctors Errors' and 'Hospital Blunders'. This is just the tip of the iceberg and no doubt there are many similar incidents that go unreported. Given the fear we have of cancer and other major life-threatening illnesses, it may surprise you to know that mistakes by doctors and hospitals are also major contributors, each year, to thousands of untimely deaths.

Standards in quality vary greatly with doctors and hospitals across the Health Service. We need to be made aware of the well-guarded fact that unnecessary deaths are, from time to time, due to misdiagnosis, negligence, incompetence, being prescribed the wrong medication or treatment and receiving care and treatment in unhygienic hospitals.

Many of us will know of a relative or friend who was admitted to hospital with a minor, certainly not a life-threatening, illness who died, without a full explanation being given to their families as to the cause of their death. The contents of this book will hopefully alert you to the dangers to watch out for, so that this doesn't happen to you or to a member of your family.

We need to be made fully aware of the importance of knowing what to do and of having the confidence in knowing how to find the best medical care and treatment for ourselves and for our families. You may also be aware of someone who had an initial diagnosis that raised little cause for concern; indeed the indication was that they had little to worry about. Unfortunately at a later date it became clear that their initial diagnosis was wrong and that their illness, which has now been diagnosed correctly, is at an advanced stage and is untreatable. This horrific situation could have been avoided if more care had been taken with the initial assessment.

We need to be clear in our minds about the state of our health and the symptoms we have and understand what to expect each time we attend

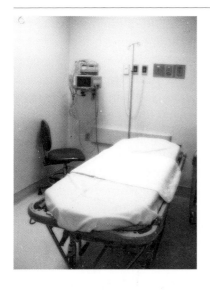

a healthcare appointment. We cannot leave our health and indeed our lives totally in the hands of doctors.

Between 20% and 25% of cancer patients are initially misdiagnosed and leave their doctor's surgery feeling relieved and thankful that they do not have a serious illness. Unfortunately, many of them are informed of the correct diagnosis at a later date when the cancer is more advanced and has spread to other organs.

Have you ever seen 'Hospital Negligence' or 'Doctor Error' cited as the cause of death on a death certificate? I bet you haven't. Important tips as to how you can safeguard your health and the health of your family are explained in this easy-to-read book.

You need to be armed with the necessary information and knowledge, in order to get the proper answers to your health questions, and to ensure that you obtain the best hea h care available.

The secrecy that surrounds mistakes made by doctors and hospitals will remain unchanged, as will information we need to know about problems that exist within the Health Service and about Health Service delivery, unless there is pressure and a demand from the public for change.

We all need to know what is happening in the Health Service. There needs to be greater openness, honesty and transparency and when mistakes are made, patients at the receiving end of these mistakes and their relatives should be told.

This should be standard practice in all hospitals. People have a right to know the truth. We, the taxpayers, are the financiers of the National Health Service. Surely receiving the best health care shouldn't be a privilege, but instead should be our collective right.

In the first couple of chapters we will take a look at the professionals who care for us – the doctors and nurses; how they are trained, what their qualifications mean and what we should expect from them. We will look at the different types of doctor, what the letters after their name actually mean and what constitutes good medical practice.

We will examine nurses, looking at Florence Nightingale and how she influenced modern nursing. We will explore the Nursing and Midwifery Council and their code and what it means for patients. The different types of nurse will be defined and their training outlined. Reference is also made to the current shortage of nurses in the NHS.

Chapter 4 looks at hospitals and how they are run. Who are the staff who will look after us during our stay? Do we have any rights? What are the responsibilities of the hospital towards us?

We look at some of the issues which affect hospital patients such as food and hospital-acquired infections such as MRSA. There is an overview of the different departments as well as information on waiting lists, budgets, equipment and hospital errors. The series of events that took place as part of the Mid Staffordshire NHS Foundation Trust scandal are reviewed.

Organisations that are linked to hospitals and the NHS such as NICE, the Care Quality Commission, the Patients Association, Monitor and the National Patient Safety Agency are explained.

The next chapter is all about the medication that we are prescribed and the medical procedures that we might need to undergo. It looks at the pharmaceutical companies and how they market drugs to the medical profession as well as how we should manage our medication and what to do about side effects.

The role of pharmacists is explained along with information about drug expiry dates and contraindications. Some of the procedures that we might need to have done are explained and your rights will be defined.

Chapter 6 is all about us as patients. The difference between being an outpatient and an inpatient, confidentiality and your choices are explained. Strategies for dealing with appointments and how to tell whether a doctor is behaving appropriately with you are all covered.

We set out the fabric of the NHS constitution and examine your

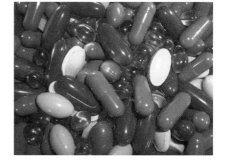

rights under it. Your responsibilities as a patient are explained and the definition of what the boundaries between doctor and patient should be.

We devote an entire chapter to children's health; covering the different age groups – babies, 1 to 5 year-olds and 6 to 15 year-olds. Their different health needs and issues are examined as well as the reviews, tests and vaccinations they will have. Going into hospital and special needs are also covered.

Pregnancy related healthcare issues are also included with information about your choices, tests you will be offered and what to expect from your midwife.

Chapter 9 compares NHS and private healthcare. The principles and structure of the NHS are set out with information on NHS Direct and the various NHS trusts. Private medical insurance is compared with the self-pay system of paying for medical treatment.

Whilst we don't want to dwell on things going wrong, it is only right that we spend a chapter looking at some of the cases where medical care has gone badly wrong. This is to raise your awareness of the types of incidents that can arise and the chain of events that can lead to disaster. The following cases are highlighted:

Robbie Powell.
Denise Hendry.
Arun Rees.
Hazel Fenton.
Dr Richard Neale.
Martin Ryan.
Emma Kemp.
Mark Cannon.
Bethany Bowen.
Penny Campbell.
Jimmy Stewart.
Lee Nicholls.
Jo Dowling.
Rosemary McFarlane.
Carla McAdam.

These will be briefly summarised with details of what went wrong with their care. An important part of dealing effectively with healthcare staff is being assertive and this is covered in chapter 11. Techniques for improving assertiveness and examples of assertive behaviour are given for you for reference purposes.

We also look at how you can ultimately take responsibility for your own health and well-being, by looking after yourself. Ideas for healthy diet and exercise are given, along with information on alternative therapies. The importance of giving up smoking is emphasised, as is the mind-body connection.

If this book saves one life, encourages one person to ask their doctor more probing questions, gets one more person to read the literature that comes with their medication, alerts one person to focus more on their health, prompts one person to research and gain a greater understanding of their medical condition, gets someone to accompany their elderly relative to an appointment with their doctor or hospital, encourages one doctor, nurse, or Health Service manager to make one small change that raises standards, prevents one medical error or one hospital mistake, then I have achieved my goal.

Life is not merely to be alive, but to be well.

Marcus Valerius Martial

Two:
Doctors

The role of the doctor is one of the most ancient professions known to the human race. Respected and revered in all cultures, to be a doctor is to hold a position of responsibility and to be looked up to by the rest of the community.

Doctors enjoy elevated social status as well as a substantial income and excellent levels of job security. Doctors are unique, in the sense, that throughout their careers, due to mistakes, medical incompetence, wrongful prescribing of medicines, botched surgery etc., a doctor may kill hundreds of patients and never be challenged about any of the deaths. They certainly appear to have 'A License To Kill'.

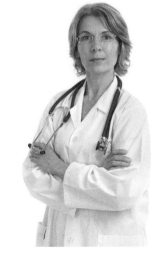

There are various different types of doctor including general practitioner (GP), surgeon, consultant and specialist. There are, however, over 50 career paths that are available to doctors. The vast majority of doctors work within the NHS, although there are opportunities within the private sector, the armed forces, the Home Office or even the prison sector.

Doctors spend many years training. They start by studying at a medical school attached to a university. To be accepted into medical school, the student should have achieved excellent results at 'A' level. During this time they will undertake clinical placements in hospitals and the community.

At the end of this period, which usually lasts for 5 years, they should graduate as a Bachelor of Medicine (BM). The degree in medicine has a core curriculum which is overseen by the GMC (General Medical Council).

All medical school graduates then have to undertake a two-year foundation programme. This was introduced in 2005 as part of the Modernising Medical Careers initiative by the NHS. The programme incorporates a series of placements which will help develop core clinical skills and a grounding in practical medicine.

This is the period when they are let loose on hospital wards and start practising on patients. It's not surprising that this period is referred to as the 'killing season'.

The final stage is called Run-Through training. This lasts for several years and is how a doctor trains in a speciality such as general practice. Once their speciality training is complete they then will be awarded a Certificate for the Completion of Training (CCT) which entitles them to be listed on the GMC's specialist register.

Once they have completed this stage they will then be required to keep up to date with developments in their specialist field by undertaking Continuing Professional Development programmes.

The whole training process can take as long as 12 years although it only takes nine years to become a GP.

There is a wide range of medical qualifications, so it is useful to know what the letters after your doctor's name signify. This is important, as later on in the book we will be looking at checking facts and making sure that the person treating you is qualified to do so. This list of qualifications can be found on page 172.

There are many wonderful doctors in the medical profession working in both the NHS as well as in private practice. Many devote their lives to the care of their patients and have saved countless lives. If you are ill, these are the doctors you need to find and if you cannot get an appointment with them as a NHS patient, then you should consider seeing them as a private patient.

As patients, we are expected to place an enormous amount of trust in doctors and so their training is extensive and their work is highly regulated. They are required to keep themselves up to date with developments in their field and to take part in educational activities throughout their career.

All doctors take an oath based on the 'Hippocratic Oath' which sets out an ethical basis for their approach to treating patients. The official documents produced by the General Medical Council, 'Duties of a Doctor' and 'Good Medical Practice', clearly state what the expectations and responsibilities should be for all doctors practising in this country. However, when mistakes are made, they close up like clams and act like a secret society, hell-bent on protecting themselves. Don't expect a doctor to give evidence against a colleague. It rarely happens.

Good Medical Practice
The Good Medical Practice guidelines require that doctors fulfil a number of criteria. They are available for all members of the public to read via the GMC website.

These include making patient care their primary concern, keeping their professional knowledge and skills up to date and making sure that they listen to patients and take their preferences and concerns into consideration.

Doctors should also give patients information if they request it and explain things in a way that they can easily understand.

It is imperative that doctors act immediately if they think that a patient may be at risk through the actions of any doctor – whether it is themselves or another.

Good Medical Practice goes on to detail specifically what patients can expect from their doctors in various areas. These include the provision of good clinical care, which encompasses adequate assessment of the patient including considering symptoms and patient history, as well as carrying out appropriate examinations.

Patients should then be offered advice or further treatment as appropriate or indeed referred to a specialist if necessary. If a patient requests a second opinion, then this request should be respected and adhered to.

The guidelines are very clear that doctors should not work beyond the limits of their competence; they should prescribe drugs only when it is absolutely certain that the medication will serve the needs of the patient and are not contraindicated by their medical history or other health issues.

The guidelines are comprehensive and do appear to set out a clear basis from which doctors should practise.

As members of society we are taught that doctors should be held in high esteem and that we should trust their opinions on what is right for us, whether that be a diagnosis or a prescribed course of treatment. Do not assume that when it comes to our health that doctors have all the answers, because they don't.

It happens that patients go to see doctors who don't have a clue as to what the proper diagnosis is and they may decide to treat them with medication for a condition the patient doesn't have. The medication could have dangerous side effects and may make the patient worse, not better.

Again, trust in their doctor has cost many patients their lives.

Unfortunately, however, what many of us fail to recognise as patients is that doctors are only human. Doctors are just as capable of being average or even below average when it comes to skills and knowledge.

Just like the rest of us they can lack motivation on some days and can make mistakes from time to time. Just like the rest of us they can come in to work with a hangover, feeling unwell or preoccupied about problems in their private life.

As we all know, this sort of thing can lead them to a lack of judgment and cause them to make mistakes. The problem is, however, that when a doctor makes a mistake it can result in illness, injury or even death. There is a saying that 'doctors bury their mistakes' which sadly turns out to be true on many occasions.

Statistics have shown that, along with cancer and heart disease, doctors are one of the three major killers in the USA.

Poor medical advice given by doctors all too often costs lives, as does incorrect treatment or, in very rare cases, deliberate mistreatment. The problem is, however, that doctors can be notoriously difficult to prosecute. Saying that though, the earliest case of a doctor being convicted of manslaughter dates back to 1831, when a woman died after giving birth.

Up until 2006, 85 doctors were charged with manslaughter, with more prosecutions taking place into the 1990s, although actual conviction rates were rather low. You have a snowball's chance in hell of successfully prosecuting a doctor.

One of the most notable cases is that of Harold Shipman who was found guilty of murdering 15 of his patients and was likely to have been responsible for as many as 218 deaths. It would seem unbelievable that someone could murder between 15 and 218 people and that their colleagues would be blind to this.

It also makes you wonder about the General Medical Council's policy to protect the public. Are doctors so busy covering their backs and the backs of their colleagues, that one of their colleagues has to kill a couple of hundred people before they even get suspicious?

At the less extreme end of the scale doctors can simply fail to give their patients the time and attention that they deserve. For example, patients often find that doctors try and rush them so that they don't get the chance to explain their symptoms fully.

Research has shown that doctors on average interrupt their patients after only 18 seconds, because they fear that the patient will 'go on and on', and that a doctor will usually make a diagnosis, in his mind, within the first 20 seconds of meeting the patient, after which he will stop listening to the patient's complaints and explanations.

According to studies, about 20% to 25% of patients seeking medical attention are misdiagnosed. This is understandable as doctors are under pressure to see more patients and to earn more money.

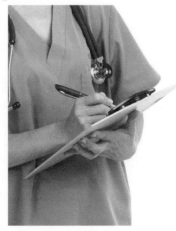

Doctors can work dangerously long hours, particularly junior hospital doctors. Surely it is impossible to make the correct decisions (which can be a matter of life or death) if you are absolutely exhausted? If a doctor is very overworked, then there is a danger that they might not devote the necessary time to your consultation and not be able to assess your symptoms fully.

Some doctors, perhaps, didn't even want to be doctors in the first place. They might have entered the profession because of family tradition or expectations and therefore just don't have the passion and motivation for the job that they would instinctively have if it had been their choice to become a doctor.

Other doctors may just have the attitude that it is just a job, and not place the importance that dealing with life and death situations truly deserves. Some doctors may even be just in the profession for the money and status.

There are a myriad of diseases, conditions, illnesses and ailments, not to mention the many drugs, treatments and therapies that are available. It is impossible for every doctor to be an expert on every single thing.

Conversely, recent implementation of European legislation means that doctors are no longer allowed to work more than 48 hours per week. This is good in some respects as it avoids situations where doctors are so exhausted that they make mistakes; however, it also means that there are more staff handovers which can put patients' lives at risk due to the lack of continuity of care.

Junior doctors working in hospitals can be a particular cause for concern, not only because they are working in a department for a relatively short period of time in order to gain experience, which can mean they do not have an in-depth knowledge of patient histories, but also because their inexperience can lead to tragedy.

Recent research from the Imperial College looked at death rates from 300,000 patients admitted to Accident and Emergency departments between 2000 and 2008 and found that patients admitted during the month of August – which is when around 50,000 junior doctors start work for the first time – are 6% more likely to die.

August has been informally dubbed 'the killing season' for some time, due to the fact that more deaths seem to occur at this time of year when the junior doctors are starting work. Similar statistics have been recorded at hospitals in the USA, with the same happening in July, which is when junior doctors start work there.

Another problem that patients can face with doctors is a language problem. The front page of the *Daily Express* reported, in March 2011, that a hospital trust expressed concerns that doctors recruited from abroad often speak such poor English that many cannot talk to their patients properly.

Imagine being treated by a doctor when there are serious communication problems. If that isn't a recipe for disaster, I don't know what is. The chairman of the NHS Foundation Trust involved stated that some of the worst English speaking doctors he had come across had been from Europe. He also claimed that some foreign locums' grasp of English was at times 'absolutely awful'.

Doctors often have an enormous amount of bureaucracy and red tape to deal with. The NHS sets targets for its staff and also has to run to increasingly tight budgets. These can be disheartening for doctors and can lead them to make inappropriate decisions.

Although many doctors now prescribe medications electronically and print out prescriptions from a computer, some still insist on handwriting prescriptions. This can lead to problems if the pharmacist cannot read their writing properly and, let's face it, doctors are notoriously bad for their impersonation of a drunken spider crawling across the prescription note.

Doctors are the most trusted of all professions. A MORI poll carried out recently showed that 92% of us think that doctors tell the truth. The survey compared a number of different professions with doctors coming out on top, with judges, clergy and scientists also scoring highly. Unsurprisingly, government ministers and journalists scored the lowest.

It is rather worrying to think that we place so much trust in other human beings who are just as fallible and capable of making mistakes as the rest of us. MORI have been carrying out this poll for 25 years, with the lowest result for doctors being 82%.

Despite this public level of trust, even the General Medical Council has been known to criticise the cultural attitude of the medical profession. In a 2001 speech, the then president of the GMC described the medical profession as a 'secretive and paternalistic culture' with a 'lack of respect' for patients.

Even the GMC guidelines require doctors to report any risks being taken by colleagues. A survey carried out by the medical website *doctors. net.uk* found that although 82% of doctors had seen their colleagues committing errors, only 15% of them had ever been reported.

As we will go on to explore later in this book, whilst doctors are definitely the right people to see when we are unwell or worried about symptoms, it is important that we retain an awareness of their fallibility and take charge of our own health issues to a major extent.

Health is not valued till sickness comes.

Dr. Thomas Fuller

Three: Nurses

At the frontline of healthcare, nurses take on many vital roles when it comes to caring for patients. The most famous nurse was Florence Nightingale who cared for injured soldiers during the Crimean War. The ideas and concepts defined by Nightingale in her book *Notes on Nursing* formed the basis for early nurse education and training.

There are more nurses in the NHS than any other type of employee. You will find them across the board in all areas of healthcare looking after every sort of person. Nurses require a degree or diploma in nursing which then enables them to register with the Nursing and Midwifery Council (NMC).

The NMC was created as a body to protect the public and to ensure that all nurses and midwives working in the UK are appropriately trained and registered. The standards required from nursing education programmes are set by the NMC and they set standards for nurses to adhere to in terms of continuing education. The NMC also has processes in place which allow for the investigation of complaints against nurses.

The Nursing and Midwifery Council has a code of conduct that all nursing staff have to abide by. The basic premise of the code is that people must be able to trust the nurse caring for them with their health and well-being. The code is then broken down into more specific requirements:

Make the care of people your first concern, treating them as individuals and respecting their dignity

Nurses should not discriminate against anyone and should treat patients with kindness and consideration at all times.

Respect people's confidentiality

Patients should be informed about how their information will be shared or used. Nurses also have a duty to disclose information if they believe that someone may be harmed otherwise.

Collaborate with those in your care

Nurses should listen to patients and respect their preferences. Efforts should be made to ensure that any language or communication barriers are surmounted. Information about their care should be shared with patients in an appropriate manner.

Ensure you gain consent

Patients should always give their consent prior to any treatment. Nurses should respect the right of patients to accept or decline treatment. They should also have an awareness of the legislation surrounding the concept of mental capacity and be able to show that they have acted in someone's best interests during an emergency.

Maintain clear professional boundaries

Nurses should not accept gifts or favours from patients that may be interpreted as a bribe; they should also not borrow or ask to borrow money from anyone in their care. There should be clear sexual barriers between nurses and patients and their families.

Work with others to protect and promote the health and well-being of those in your care, their families and carers, and the wider community

Share information with your colleagues

Nurses should pass on relevant patient information to others involved in your care. They should also work with one another to monitor their standards of care. Students should be facilitated wherever possible.

Work effectively as part of a team
Respect colleagues, take advice and share skills as appropriate. Make referrals if necessary.

Delegate effectively
If nurses delegate they must ensure that their instructions can be carried out, that there is help and support available and that the outcome is successful.

Manage risk
If a nurse believes that someone is at risk because of the practices of themselves or others then they must take action immediately. If it is not possible to meet the standards of the code then a senior staff member must be informed immediately. Concerns should be put in writing.

Provide a high standard of practice and care at all times

Use the best available evidence
Care and advice should be based on the best evidence available.

Keep your skills and knowledge up to date
Nurses should work within the levels of their competence and keep their knowledge and practical skills up to date by participating in learning activities.

Keep clear and accurate records
Records should be updated as soon as possible after an event, they should not be tampered with, and they should also be legible. Everything should be signed, dated and timed and kept securely.

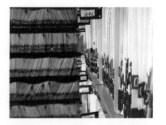

Be open and honest, act with integrity and uphold the reputation of your profession
Nurses should demonstrate their commitment to equality and diversity. They should adhere to the law and keep the NMC informed about any criminal records. If their fitness to practise is in doubt they should inform their employer.

Deal with problems

Respond truthfully to complaints and do not prejudice the care of someone who may have complained. If a patient suffers harm, a nurse should act immediately by explaining everything to the patient. Nurses should always cooperate with investigations.

Be impartial

Nurses should not use their status to promote non-health related causes. They should protect the confidentiality of patients if dealing with the media.

There are different types of nurses:

Adult nurses

This type of nurse can be found in hospitals or in the community, working with adults of all ages.

Mental Health nurses

Mental Health nurses specialise in caring for patients with mental health conditions ranging from schizophrenia to depression.

Children's nurses

This type of nurse looks after children from babies to teenagers in a variety of settings.

Learning Disability nurses

Learning Disability nurses work in both residential and community settings caring for people with learning disabilities.

District Nurses

District Nurses undergo further postgraduate training to qualify as specialist practitioners. They then work with patients in the community who have a variety of conditions.

Neonatal nursing

This is a specialist branch of nursing which involves caring for premature babies. The training is undertaken by those who have already qualified as registered nurses or midwives.

Health Visitors
Registered nurses or midwives undergo further specialist training to work with families in many different settings.

Practice nurses
Practice nurses work within GP surgeries and take on a range of responsibilities including giving vaccinations and contraceptive advice.

Prison nurses
As the title suggests, this nurse works within a prison setting, where patients are often struggling with mental health issues and drug addiction. This makes for a varied and challenging role.

School nurses
Working within a school setting, this sort of nursing focuses on children and is usually only open to experienced registered nurses.

Nurse training
In order to become a nurse it is necessary to study for a degree or diploma in nursing. Courses specialise in one of the four main areas of nursing:

Adult.
Child.
Mental Health.
Learning Disabilities.

A full-time degree takes three years to complete although it is also possible to study nursing on a part-time basis. The degree begins with the Common Foundation Programme (CFP) which acts as an all-round introduction to nursing, covering aspects of all four main nursing fields, as well as maternity care.

The nursing diploma follows a similar pattern, but requires fewer credits to be achieved. Nurses with a diploma can register, begin working and then undertake additional study and training to achieve degree level.

Half of the programme is based around supervised nursing in practice. Student nurses work both in hospitals and the community. 12

or 18 months are spent on the CFP with 18 or 24 months in one of the specialist nursing areas.

Nurse shortages and standards of care

There has been a well-publicised shortage of nurses in the UK for many years now. The Royal College of Nursing has released figures which suggest that nurses themselves feel that patient care is being compromised regularly as a consequence of staff shortages. The 2009 Employment Survey asked 9,000 nurses a range of questions, with 55% of respondents saying that they felt that they were 'too busy to provide the level of care they would like' and 67% felt that their workload was too heavy.

However, there cannot be any excuses for low standards of nursing care. It has been reported in the media, on more than one occasion, of elderly patients being neglected, for example, being dehydrated, not being fed their meals, not being properly washed and being discovered to have been lying in urine and faeces.

These low standards of nursing care cannot be justified, nor should they be tolerated. It cannot be explained away by crying about staff shortages, as hundreds of other hospitals throughout the UK have the same levels of staffing and similar budgets, yet they provide their patients with high standards of nursing care.

One of the problems is that nursing staff do not spend enough time with their patients, the reason being that they spend too much time writing reports and adding statistics to a computer. Hospital wards would benefit from more efficient, streamlined and better management.

In other words, bring back the old style ward sisters and matrons and prune the existing management structures. Patients and their relatives have to accept some of the responsibility for low standards of care, as they are too accepting of what is given to them and they don't complain often enough or loudly enough.

Health is worth more than learning.

Thomas Jefferson

Four:
Hospitals

Most people have to visit a hospital at some point during their lives. Many visits are straightforward and routine, such as attending for blood tests and other types of outpatient appointment. Others can be more significant, such as having to go into hospital for an operation, for treatment or to Accident and Emergency.

Regardless of the reason for your visit to hospital, it is important to be aware of some key facts and to remember the choices and rights that are available to you.

There are many different types of hospitals, some are large and others are small; some are private and others are run by the NHS. Certain hospitals specialise in particular medical conditions, but all hospitals operate on the basic premise of being a place to care for patients.

General hospitals are usually large with numerous departments dealing with a variety of different specialities. Many major cities have specialist children's hospitals. There are a number of psychiatric hospitals in the UK also. Teaching hospitals are linked to a medical school.

The sort of departments found within hospitals include Accident and Emergency, a burns unit, cardiology, neurology, intensive care, oncology, gynaecology and obstetrics, maternity, physiotherapy, pathology and X-ray.

The staff is varied according to the department but some work in more than one area.

Accident and Emergency (A&E)

Also known as Casualty, this is where ambulances take patients in an emergency situation although you can also make your own way there if you have had an accident. Staffed 24 hours a day, patients are usually assessed by a triage nurse and then treated according to the urgency of their condition.

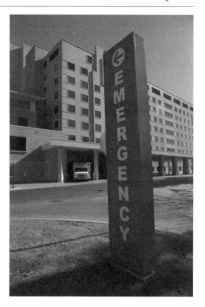

Anaesthetics

This department is responsible for providing anaesthetics to patients undergoing surgery. They can also assist with pain relief for short or long-term conditions and for women in labour.

Breast screening

Usually linked to the X-ray department, women can come here for mammograms which check for signs of breast cancer.

Cardiology

Patients who have conditions of the heart or circulation are treated here on an inpatient or outpatient basis.

Chaplaincy

Along with the hospital chapel, the hospital chaplains are there to provide spiritual and emotional support to patients and their relatives.

Intensive Care Unit (ICU)

Also known as Critical Care, this is where patients who are very seriously ill are looked after on an intensive basis by specialist staff.

X-ray

Sometimes now referred to as Diagnostic Imaging, this department performs all types of X-rays and scans including ultrasound, CT and MRI scanning.

Discharge lounge

This is where patients can go just before they return home from the hospital. They will still have access to medical services but can relax and readjust before leaving the hospital.

Ear, Nose and Throat

This department looks after patients with conditions affecting these parts of the body.

Elderly services

Elderly people suffer from a range of unique problems and conditions. This department specialises in their needs.

Gastroenterology

Conditions related to the bowels, intestines, pancreas and bile duct are treated by the specialist staff in this department.

General surgery

General surgery can cover all types of procedures including appendix removal, tonsils removal and gallbladder removal.

Gynaecology

This department specialises in female reproductive and urinary conditions.

Haematology

In conjunction with the hospital laboratories, this department oversees patients suffering from blood diseases and problems.

Maternity

This department provides care to women during pregnancy and childbirth.

Microbiology

The staff in this department test samples from patients for different types of infection.

Neonatal Unit

Babies who require specialist care due to prematurity or illness are cared for here by specialist staff.

Nephrology

Patients with kidney problems are treated in this department. Services such as dialysis are offered and staff liaise with the transplant team on behalf of patients.

Neurology

Disorders of the nervous system, such as brain and spinal conditions can be treated here.

Nutrition and Dietetics

This department works in conjunction with other specialities to provide nutritional advice to patients.

Obstetrics and Gynaecology

This department offers maternity services and specialist care relating to pregnancy.

Occupational Therapy

This department works in conjunction with others to provide physical and mental therapy to patients.

Oncology

Cancer patients are treated in this department with treatments such as radiotherapy and chemotherapy.

Ophthalmology

This department deals with specialist eye diagnosis, testing and treatment for adults and children.

Orthopaedics

Anything to do with bones and muscles is treated here.

Pain Management Clinics
These are usually run by consultant anaesthetists for people suffering from long-term pain.

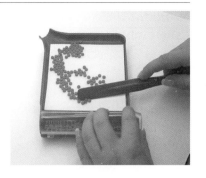

Pharmacy
The hospital pharmacy is responsible for administering the medication throughout the hospital.

Physiotherapy
Physiotherapists often work closely with the orthopaedic team to treat patients who need help with movement and manipulation after surgery or injury.

Radiotherapy
This is a form of X-ray treatment for cancer.

Renal unit
The renal unit is closely linked to nephrology and provides haemodialysis treatment.

Rheumatology
Musculoskeletal disorders are treated by this department.

Sexual health
Also known as genitourinary medicine, this department helps with sexually transmitted infections, as well as family planning care.

Urology
Kidney and bladder problems are treated in this department.

(Source: Henderson, 2008)

Generally speaking, larger hospitals are in a position to offer the best service and treatment options. They usually have access to a much larger budget, which makes it possible for them to employ more senior and experienced staff and to purchase better equipment.

It is surprising to note that when, sadly, patients die in hospital, approximately 20% of hospital deaths are due to factors other than the illness or condition that the patient was hospitalised for.

Statistics show also that 1 in every 6 hospital patients has actually been made ill by a doctor. In the USA there are many thousands of deaths every year which have been caused by hospital errors.

Hospital infections

There are, quite rightly, very big concerns about the large number of hospital infections with so-called 'superbugs' like MRSA and C. dif which are frequently mentioned in the news. If these types of infection are to be avoided then it is essential that cleanliness and hygiene are top priority in the hospital.

If, as a patient, you see any evidence that these areas are lacking then you must complain immediately. Figures released by the Office for National Statistics in August 2009 showed that around 30,000 people had died from these two infections inside a five-year period. This is about three times as many deaths as occur on the roads every year.

The front page headline in the *Belfast Telegraph* on 22 March 2011 was 'Dirty wards cost 31 lives'. Findings of an independent probe into an outbreak of Clostridium difficile in the Northern Health and Social Care Trust hospitals found the superbug played a part in 31 deaths between June 2007 and August the following year.

Evidence highlighted hygiene failures at Antrim Area Hospital. The inquiry reported 'startling lapses in basic hygiene' and the distressing and often humiliating experiences of those who contracted C. dif. It is

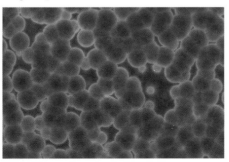

claimed that superbugs have contributed to the deaths of 459 people in Northern Ireland in the last six years.

Certainly the advancement of time doesn't always equate with progress. During the 1960s and 1970s, matrons and ward sisters made sure that wards were spotlessly clean and standards of care were high. They would be shocked and horrified by the dirty wards and low standards of care that exist today and which are brought to our attention, by the media, on a regular basis.

MRSA, which stands for Methicillin-Resistant Staphylococcus Aureus, generally occurs in people who are already unwell and usually in the hospital. It is notoriously difficult to treat because the bacteria that cause the illness are resistant to antibiotics. It can lead to serious conditions such as septicaemia, pneumonia, osteomyelitis and endocarditis. Generalised MRSA screening was introduced for most hospital patients prior to admission in March 2009.

Leslie Ash

Well known actress, Leslie Ash, was unfortunate enough to contract MRSA. She was awarded £5,000,000 in compensation by the NHS Litigation Authority and will have to take painkillers for the rest of her life. The amount of compensation awarded was the highest ever in the case of a hospital-acquired infection.

The actress contracted a strain of MRSA at the Chelsea and Westminster Hospital after being admitted with a punctured lung and two broken ribs. The infection is thought to have come from an epidural needle which came loose. An abscess developed which put pressure on her spinal cord and brought her very close to death. Her children had to be told that she might not survive. She spent several months partially paralysed as a result of the condition.

She has joined forces with the Patients Association to help improve hygiene in hospitals and is also helping to promote a campaign by the University of Nottingham to raise money to fund research by scientists at the Centre for Healthcare Associated Infections (CHAI) into ways of preventing and treating these infections.

CHAI is a joint effort by nine different academic schools at the University of Nottingham, as well as Nottingham University Hospitals

NHS Trust. The research programme is working to develop new vaccines and antibiotics, also on methods to detect and identify strains of C. difficile. They are developing new methods of testing for MRSA and carrying out work to help them understand exactly how C. difficile spreads within a hospital environment.

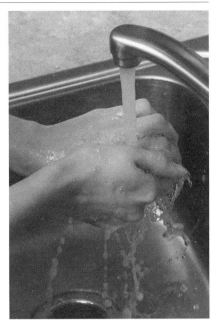

Clostridium difficile, also known as C. dif., is another serious antibiotic-resistant infection. It is most common in people who have recently taken a course of antibiotics and usually occurs in patients in a hospital environment.

There are a number of measures that can be taken to ensure that infection rates are minimised, and these include hand washing and sanitisation.

Unfortunately, however, a recent audit carried out for NHS Lothian showed that 1 in 5 senior doctors and consultants failed to wash their hands between patients. In 2006, Lothian was identified as the worst area in Scotland for C. dif. related deaths, when over 40 patients died in the space of a single year.

Lothian is not alone however. The Regulation and Quality Improvement Authority assessed hospitals in Northern Ireland during 2009 and found that 8 out of 19 areas inspected were below the minimum levels recommended for hand hygiene, clinical practice, equipment and environment.

The Care Quality Commission, which came into existence in early 2009, found that 21 out of the 288 NHS trusts registered with them also failed to meet hygiene standards.

These worrying statistics make it no surprise that superbug infections are still occurring and still causing unnecessary pain, suffering and even death. If you are in hospital and see evidence of poor hygiene then you should make a complaint as soon as possible.

Waiting lists

Waiting lists are an ongoing problem in the NHS. Sadly some patients have had to wait so long for an operation that they have actually died before it could be carried out.

Since 2008 it has been the aim of the NHS to ensure that all patients having been referred for treatment receive their treatment within 18 weeks.

Being on a hospital waiting list can cause a patient to have to spend more time in the hospital. It can also be very worrying to have to spend a long time waiting for treatment. Any pain and discomfort that the patient is suffering has to be endured whilst being on the waiting list.

There is concern, however, that European laws which have come into force regulating the number of hours that doctors can work will have a negative effect on the amount of operations that can take place, meaning that patients may have to wait even longer for their treatment.

Budgets

The NHS is infamous for having to stick to budgets and reach specific performance targets. Unfortunately though, this is all too often at the expense of patients' well-being. Patients who could benefit from an expensive drug or treatment are frequently not given the opportunity because their NHS Trust will not fund the treatment.

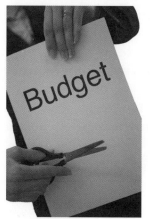

The cost of drugs is a major concern as expensive medicines are increasingly stretching hospital budgets. Recent figures released by Audit Scotland showed that the bill for drugs in Scottish hospitals had increased by 76% over the preceding 5 years. This equates to £70 per hospital patient per year.

The figures for Scotland showed that drug spending had increased more than any other hospital related spending.

In general, hospitals are in a budgetary crisis, even though nearly £90 billion had been spent on the NHS in 2010.

This means that there is a shortfall which will prevent future improvements and investments going ahead as planned. Only five hospital trusts have achieved an underspend.

Most NHS trusts will have to look at cost cutting measures including reducing the number of staff they employ, freezing recruitment, postponing operations, and delaying payment to suppliers. None of these measures can possibly have anything other than a negative impact on patient care.

From April 2010 the Care Quality Commission will have greater powers to enforce the standards required from NHS hospitals. They will be able to prosecute, issue fines and even de-register trusts which fail to perform.

NHS patients can make the choice as to where and when they receive hospital treatment. The Dr Foster Hospital Guide is a comprehensive directory of NHS and private hospitals which you can use to compare waiting times and infection rates from MRSA and C. dif., alongside other relevant information to help you make the right choice of hospital for you.

Parking

Another issue which affects hospital patients is parking. Recently, many hospital trusts have come under fire for the exorbitant parking fees that most patients and visitors are subjected to. Many people feel that the costs are an unjustified tax on the sick.

According to the NHS Information Centre some hospitals charge as much as £5.10 for three hours parking. 32% of hospitals make a charge for parking on the premises. If the hospital that you need to attend does charge for parking then it is worth checking whether the hospital offers a concession scheme for people who need to park there regularly. Hospitals have been urged to provide free parking for patients undergoing chemotherapy or renal treatment as these procedures typically take several hours over which time parking fees can build up quite considerably.

Food and nutrition

Food is important to all of us, and particularly to those who are unwell or recovering from an illness.

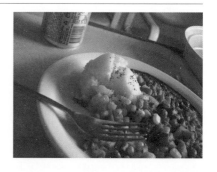

Most hospitals serve three meals a day, breakfast, lunch and dinner, while operating a menu card system whereby patients can make their food choices for the following day by ticking selections on a card which is distributed to them. Special dietary needs are usually catered for by prior arrangement. Some hospitals are also now offering the option of snack boxes which enable patients to graze at their leisure.

One might expect the food in hospital to be of the highest standard and to be of top nutritional quality. Unfortunately this is not always the case. The amount spent per patient on food per day varies wildly between the different NHS hospital trusts. The average spent per patient per day is £7.43, with the lowest being just £2.80 and the highest £18.20.

This means that the food standard and quality in hospitals will vary according to which trust you are dealing with. There are plans in place to ensure that hospitals take patient satisfaction into consideration much more. Patients will be asked to complete satisfaction surveys about the food they have been served and, if the hospital fails to meet the targets set for it, then their budget will be cut or they will be sanctioned in other ways.

An Internet blogger known as Traction Man recently highlighted the poor quality of hospital food when he posted a series of photographs on his blog of the food he had been served in hospital whilst suffering from osteomyelitis. He devised the series as a game called Hospital Food Bingo and encouraged his readers to guess what was on the plate. The interest garnered by this blogger raised the issue of hospital food and its poor quality. Followers of the blog failed to identify around half of the dishes photographed.

Researchers from Bournemouth University studied food served by NHS hospitals and compared it with the menu on offer to prison inmates. Their findings showed that prison food had an excellent nutritional content.

Patients in hospital, even when served with good food, faced obstacles when it actually came to eating it. The researchers found that assistance with eating was often not offered and that staff did not monitor patients to ensure that they were eating well. Trays are often removed by cleaning staff before the medical team has had a chance to assess what the patient has eaten.

The Patient Environment Action Team monitors the food served in hospitals and awards star ratings so that patients can know what to expect in terms of food during their stay in hospital.

There have been recorded incidences of patients having to order takeaway food to their bedside because of the lack of suitable meals for them in the hospital.

If you are facing a stay in the hospital and you are concerned about the food, then it is a good idea to contact the hospital and ask them to provide you with a typical menu card so you can get an idea of what you will be served with whilst you are a patient. You could try contacting PALS (Patient Advice and Liaison Service) for more information.

Food, or rather the lack of it, also contributes to hospital deaths. Statistics show that over 240 patients every year die of starvation whilst in hospital. If, whilst in hospital, you have any cause for concern about food or feeding issues then it is imperative that they are raised with nursing staff as soon as possible. Don't leave it too late for things to be rectified.

The Mid Staffordshire NHS Foundation Trust scandal
The Mid Staffordshire NHS Foundation Trust was highlighted as a shocking example of failings in patient care. A third inquiry has been launched into the events here after as many as 1,200 patients died because of failings in care standards.

Examples of failures included using reception staff to carry out initial checks on patients being admitted, heart monitors being turned off because nurses were not aware of how to use them, insufficient staffing levels, no routine discussion of care quality and a lack of night time cover.

Although patients and their relatives had been complaining to the NHS trust for some time, their complaints were not being acted upon which allowed the failings to go on unchecked for much longer than they should have done. It was only when the Healthcare Commission noticed that death rates at the hospital were much higher than they should have been that investigations started to take place.

Many patients died needlessly. One had been left for three days with an untreated fracture in their thighbone and another contracted C. difficile and was left for four hours in a soiled bed. Visitors to the hospital reported seeing patients drinking out of flower vases because they were so thirsty and that wards and bathrooms were dirty and unhygienic.

Conditions at the hospital were described as being like something from the Third World. The problems were compounded by the fact that there was a closed culture in place which dissuaded staff from raising concerns about failings and poor standards.

The report into the investigation carried out by the Healthcare Commission was published in March 2009. The report focused on emergency admissions, for which the trust seemed to have an abnormally high death rate. The Accident and Emergency Department was found to be understaffed and lacking in essential equipment.

Patients frequently had to wait for pain relief and for wounds to be dressed. There were frequently no senior doctors on duty in the hospital after 9pm, leaving only inexperienced juniors to cope on their own.

Standards of cleanliness were so poor that patients were being left for extended periods of time with wet or soiled sheets and wards and bathrooms were not being cleaned. Patient observations were not taken regularly with staff failing to spot when deteriorations were occurring in the condition of patients, or if deterioration was identified, with no action being taken.

The report identified the key areas in which the trust was failing and earmarked them as areas in which the trust needed to improve its performance. At the time, no organisation was in a position to impose any sort of sanction on the trust for failing patients on such a large scale.

Hospitals under pressure
'NHS reforms: Hospitals under pressure. Waiting lists are growing, more operations are being cancelled and treatment is being rationed. At least 20,000 doctors and nurses are to be cut'. These articles appeared in *The Independent* in April 2011.

It's fairly obvious that this is not going to reduce doctors' errors or hospital blunders, quite the opposite. 'The number of emergency operations cancelled by hospitals in England has risen by a quarter in the past seven months.' 'Growing numbers of patients are having to wait for more than four hours to be seen in casualty departments, and the proportion who still had no bed four hours after being admitted doubled between April and December'.

The way the Health Service is heading doesn't exactly fill you with confidence, does it? It seems that, when financial pressures hit the NHS, it is frontline services to patients that always bear the brunt. The NHS managers don't appear to go overboard cutting management jobs and bureaucracy. No, that wouldn't get the same publicity from the media and pressure the Government for more funding. Do they ever put the patient first?

NICE

The National Institute for Health and Clinical Excellence (NICE) produces guidance on the prevention and treatment of ill health as well as the promotion of good health.

It is responsible for making the decisions on what drugs and treatments are made available on the NHS. They use a complex calculation to determine the improvement in the patient's quality of life that the treatment will offer, as well as the extra extension of life that will benefit the patient.

This is then compared with the drugs and therapies already in existence and already being used, and a decision is made by weighing up these various different factors. The decisions are made independently of budgetary considerations as there are already NHS trusts that have started to ration the treatment available so that they do not go over budget.

The guidelines are then made available for healthcare professionals and patients to refer to on the NICE website – *nice.org.uk*. Each condition (i.e. depression, diabetes and so on) has its own clinical guideline which recommends the sort of care and support that should be available and the treatments and drug therapies that are available.

Doctors can use the guidelines as a frame of reference to ensure that they are recommending treatment and prescribing drugs correctly. Patients can also access the information so that they have a full awareness of what the NHS can offer them in relation to their condition.

Hospital staff
Whilst in hospital you will come into contact with various different staff members, which can be more than a little bit confusing.

Doctors
Doctors in hospitals usually fall into one of the following categories:

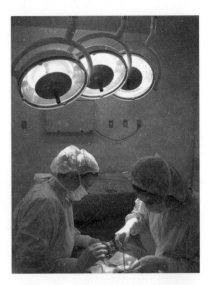

Consultant Surgeon
The consultant is in charge of your overall care and works with a team of doctors. You might see your consultant when you attend an outpatient appointment and they might see you whilst carrying out ward rounds, but they may not carry out your actual operation.

Specialist Surgical Registrar
Most surgeons work in this role for around six years under the supervision of a consultant. They eventually choose an area in which they intend to specialise, prior to completing their training and becoming a consultant.

Senior House Officer
SHOs work under the supervision of a consultant and are learning how to carry out surgery and gaining experience of carrying out the various surgical procedures.

Associate Specialist Surgeon
Working under the supervision of a consultant, this type of doctor is responsible for lots of different aspects of surgical care.

Staff Grade Surgeon

After having gained some experience as a registrar, these doctors often alternate on the emergency surgical rota. Their work is supervised by a consultant.

Pre-registration House Officer

Newly qualified doctors spend a year in this role prior to becoming eligible for registration with the GMC. They usually spend six months in a surgical role and six months in general medicine.

There are also, for example, consultant physicians and registrar physicians as well as consultants and registrars for all other specialist fields, such as dermatology, ENT and so on.

Doctors that you may come across in hospital may be students or be fully qualified. They may be referred to as Dr, or if they carry out surgery, Mr, Mrs, or Ms. Some doctors have achieved Professor status and are referred to in this way.

Medical students

They can be at varying stages of their 5-year medical degree.

Junior Doctors

Having completed their medical degree, they are still undergoing training towards becoming a Consultant or GP. There are four different grades:

Foundation Year 1.
Foundation Year 2.
GP Registrar.
Speciality Registrar.

Senior Doctors

They have completed their training. Senior Doctor job titles are:

Consultant.
GP.

Staff Doctor.
Speciality Doctor.
Associate Specialist.
Trust Doctor.
Hospital Practitioner.
Clinical Assistant.
Clinical Medical Officer.

They are also referred to as staff and associate specialists (or SAS doctors).

Academic Doctors
They are fully qualified doctors who teach or carry out research and also practice. Job titles include:

Clinical Academic Fellow.
Clinical Lecturer.
Clinical Research Fellow.
Lecturer.
Senior Lecturer.
Professor.
Reader.

There are a number of other specialist doctors such as:

Anaesthetist - responsible for anaesthetics during operations and pain relief services.
Emergency Medicine Doctor - specialises in Accident and Emergency work.
Gynaecologist - specialises in the female reproductive system.
Obstetrician - provides specialist care for women during pregnancy and childbirth.
Occupational Physician - treats conditions related to industrial environments.
Opthalmologist - specialises in eye disorders.
Paediatrician - looks after children and babies.

Pathologist - diagnoses diseases by studying tissue samples.
Cardiologist - specialises in the heart, arteries and veins.
Dermatologist - treats skin conditions.
Endocrinologist - treats hormone related conditions.
Gastroenterologist - specialises in diseases of the digestive tract.
Geriatrician - cares for elderly patients.
Haematologist - specialises in conditions related to the blood.
Neurologist - treats disorders of the nervous system.
Oncologist - specialises in treating cancer patients.
Renal Physician - also known as a nephrologist, specialises in the kidneys.
Respirologist - specialises in the treatment of lung disorders.
Rheumatologist - treats arthritis and related conditions.
Psychiatrist - specialises in the treatment of mental disorders.
Public Health Doctor - works with disease in populations.
Radiologist - is trained to interpret images of the body such as X-rays and ultrasound scans.

Apart from doctors, you may also come into contact with other types of healthcare staff such as:

Nurses
Nurses can be found throughout hospitals, working in many different settings. Depending on whether they specialise in a particular field, they can be found working with people of all ages who have lots of different health issues.

Hospital pharmacists
They work closely with medical staff to advise on medication for all kinds of patients. They also dispense medication within the pharmacy and prepare drugs that need to be tailor-made such as certain cancer treatments.

Midwives
Midwives work closely with women before, during and after childbirth.

Health Visitors
Specialising in the needs of children under five, Health Visitors are qualified nurses with at least two years experience post-registration.

Physiotherapists
Physiotherapists work with patients of all ages who are suffering from movement related issues.

Radiographers
There are two types of Radiographer – diagnostic and therapeutic:

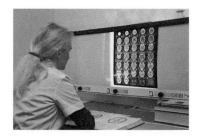

Diagnostic Radiographers work with X-rays, CT Scans, MRI Scans and Ultrasound to take images of the inside of the body to assist in diagnosis.

Therapeutic Radiographers work with cancer patients, delivering controlled doses of radiation as a treatment for the disease.

Podiatrists
Also known as chiropodists, they specialise in the lower leg and foot, treating ailments and injuries on people of all ages.

Speech and Language Therapists
Speech and Language Therapists work with patients who have difficulties with their speech or with chewing and swallowing.

Counsellors
Counselling is a 'talking therapy' which can be useful in a wide range of situations.

Occupational Therapists
Occupational Therapists use a range of activities to help treat physical and mental conditions.

Psychologists

Psychologists are not medically qualified. However they specialise in how the mind works and can be found in a number of settings.

Non-medical staff that you may encounter in hospital include:

Porters

Porters play a vital role in transporting patients and specialist equipment around the hospital and between departments.

ICT staff

There is a vast amount of technology at work in a typical hospital and the ICT staff will be on hand to ensure that everything is set up correctly and functions as it should.

Clinical Manager

They are responsible for ensuring that everything required to deliver care to patients is all running as it should.

Caterers

Most hospitals will have a large catering team who are in charge of making sure that all patients are fed with a nutritionally balanced diet during their stay in hospital.

Equipment

Whilst many hospitals are extremely well equipped with the most up to date equipment for treating their patients, figures from the Taxpayers Alliance suggest that many hospitals are simply not making use of the often sophisticated technology that is available to them.

One example is the use of linear accelerators which are used to treat cancer. It is recommended by the National Radiotherapy Advisory Group that each machine should be delivering about 8,000 doses every year, but on average only 7,191 doses are actually

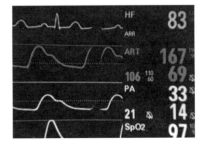

being administered. Some trusts were found to be delivering as few as 5,000 doses per machine.

The report calculated that if all machines were being used to their full capacity then an additional 128,000 doses could be given every year which is the same as having 18 more machines.

Some of the machinery and equipment that you might expect to find in hospital includes Computerised Tomography (CT) Scanners, Magnetic Resonance Imagery (MRI) Scanners and Heart-lung machines.

Theft in hospitals

Unfortunately sometimes equipment goes astray, which means that some hospitals have to depend on WiFi tagging to keep track of the whereabouts of their expensive devices. There have also been many incidences of medical equipment being stolen by criminals.

Some items have been taken 'to order' by specialist criminal gangs and others have been taken by opportunists. Computers and laptops are frequently stolen which can lead to breaches of confidential patient records data. More than 522 laptops alone have been stolen from hospital wards over a 3-year period. Examples of thefts include cardiovascular equipment, worth £78,000, stolen from Addenbrookes Hospital in Cambridgeshire; £114,000 worth of gastrology equipment going missing from the Royal Hallamshire Hospital and ultrasound machines worth £41,000 from West Middlesex University Hospital.

Arrowe Park Hospital in the Wirral had eight hospital beds stolen which cost over £4,000 to replace and 800 units of Botox were stolen from York Hospital which were worth £3,000. This type of crime has forced some hospitals to divert money away from patient care to be invested in security systems such as CCTV. There is a market for stolen medical equipment abroad.

Hospital errors

The number of hospital beds available to patients in the UK is less than in other parts of Europe. The UK has just 388 beds per 100,000 population, compared with 870 in Germany, 720 in France and 640 in Belgium.

Figures released in January 2009 showed that patient deaths as a result of hospital mistakes had increased by 60% in the preceding two years.

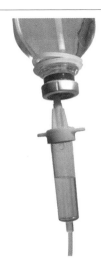

At least 3,645 patients died because of hospital-acquired infections, mistakes during operations, incorrect diagnoses, wrongly administered drugs and faulty medical equipment. Others died because of abuse by staff or visitors, or due to issues arising from being transferred to different wards or other hospitals.

Errors can occur due to lack of staff or overcrowding of wards. Known as Serious Untoward Incidents (SUIs), errors frequently go unreported or are not reported to their full extent. It has been recorded that the NHS has paid out around £4 million since 2004 in compensation to patients who had undergone operations on the incorrect part of their bodies.

Another common error relates to the administering of injections. Statistics show that patients are all too frequently given the wrong dose or even the wrong drug and sometimes the drug is administered via the wrong route or given at the wrong time.

The mistakes occur, according to the research, because of staff stress or tiredness, heavy workload, change of drug names, or lack of experience and supervision.

There is hope, however. Hospital pharmacist, Margaret Ledger-Scott, recently won an award for improving patient safety. She came up with the idea for a scheme whereby patients are issued with a 'Healthcare book' within which all their treatment is recorded.

During a trial, the use of her scheme saw medication errors drop from 72% to only 2%. The scheme is being used in the North East region and will hopefully be rolled out to other parts of the UK in the future. Ms Ledger-Scott was quoted as saying that 'it is really about involving patients as the number one person in the care process.... It is about making them aware that errors can be made and empowering them to have control over their own medication'.

Sadly, some incidents that occur in hospitals which affect patient well-being or survival are due to criminal behaviour and not simple errors. The case of Beverly Allitt hit the headlines a few years ago after she killed several patients.

There are a number of organisations in existence that can offer information, support and advice when it comes to hospitals and healthcare in general.

Care Quality Commission

This organisation has been put in place to regulate health and social care services in England. They assess and regulate hospitals and from April 2010 have had the power to prosecute and issue fines against hospitals that are not meeting required standards of care, service and hygiene.

If you want to find out more about the hospital that you are going to be attending, then their website offers a service to enable you to find and compare your local services, so you know what to expect and have the information you need to make decisions about where you have your treatment. There are results of surveys from patients and staff to give you a more in-depth picture of what the service is offering to patients.

Patients Association

This organisation was created over 40 years ago in order to represent the needs of the patient in healthcare. It is a registered charity and encourages patients to share their experiences of the NHS by using the information to then work with NHS providers to help improve the services they offer.

They receive no funding from the Department of Health and are an independent organisation. They campaign on behalf of many healthcare related causes and produce regular reports. They can offer independent help and advice on many healthcare related issues and operate a telephone helpline. They produce a number of advice booklets as well as a quarterly magazine. If you have a healthcare issue that you think needs looking at, then they are an excellent organisation to contact.

Monitor

Monitor is the independent regulator for NHS Foundation Trusts. Established in 2004, Monitor is directly accountable to parliament. They are responsible for establishing the readiness of a trust to become a Foundation Trust (FT), ensuring that Foundation Trusts comply with the conditions of their status as FT, and to support the development of NHS Foundation Trusts.

When assessing trusts for foundation status they examine a number of different aspects including whether the trust is able to operate efficiently, economically and effectively, whether the trust is capable of meeting healthcare targets and adhering to national standards, and ensuring that the trust is able to cooperate effectively with other NHS trusts.

Monitor then checks, on a regular basis, that the trust is continuing to comply with all of the necessary requirements and recommends appropriate courses of action where necessary.

National Patient Safety Agency
The National Patient Safety Agency (NPSA) is what is known as an 'Arms Length Body' of the Department of Health. It is split into three divisions:

National Reporting and Learning Service
NRLS reports on patient safety incidents and works to identify avoidable risks.

National Clinical Assessment Service
NCAS works with healthcare organisations to resolve concerns about the performance of individuals such as doctors and dentists.

National Research Ethics Service
NRES monitors clinical trials taking place in the UK and works to protect the participants.

The National Patient Safety Agency also monitors:

National Confidential Inquiry into Suicide and Homicide by People with Mental Illness
This body examines all incidents of suicide and homicide by people in contact with mental health services, with a view to reducing the risks of similar incidents in the future.

Confidential Enquiry into Maternal and Child Health
This is a registered charity which aims to improve the health of mothers and their children through research.

National Confidential Enquiry into Patient Outcome and Death
This aims to improve standards of care for patients by reviewing patient management.

A man too busy to take care of his health is like a mechanic too busy to take care of his tools.

Spanish Proverb

Five: Medication and Procedures

Most of us need to take some form of medication at some time in our lives. There are a wide variety of drugs available to us, both over the counter and on prescription. The correct medication can combat infection or help manage a long-term condition. It is essential, however, that medication 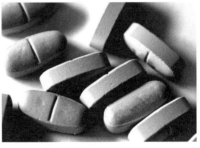 is used in the right way, that it is prescribed under the right circumstances and that its use is regularly reviewed.

It is important to remember that any sort of drug is effectively a poison that can kill you if it is not used in the right way. There are 7,000 deaths every year from drug errors. Even junior doctors can write prescriptions for very dangerous medications, and there is concern over the lack of training in this area. The General Medical Council has been reviewing the issue after a survey carried out two years ago found that medical students were 'very concerned about their ability to prescribe'.

Leading pharmacologist, Professor David Webb of Edinburgh University, appeared before the Commons Health Select Committee to outline concerns about the instruction given to junior doctors in this area.

(Source: BBC News, 2009)

New drugs and new treatments are emerging at such a rate that it would not be possible to expect any doctor to be totally competent with every one of them. Even a highly motivated doctor, with a busy schedule, would not have the time to keep fully up to date with everything that comes on the market. Again, our research could prove to be most valuable and any treatment that you feel may be relevant to your condition should, by all means, be brought to the attention of your doctor.

Manage your medication

If you are prescribed a drug, take some time to read the instructions and check the expiry date. Read the section about contraindications and side effects carefully in case there is something that your doctor has missed or forgotten to mention to you.

Be proactive about your medication. When you see your doctor, make sure that you are very clear about your symptoms. Also, if you are seeing more than one doctor, make sure that they all know what medications you are taking. You are the best judge of whether it is helping you or not and you are not obliged to accept the opinion of the doctors treating you.

If you are prescribed a drug, then do question your doctor about it. You are entitled to know whether this is a tried and tested medication or whether it is a new product that hasn't been available for very long. If you are taking part in an experiment then you want to know about it.

You could perhaps ask your doctor to describe some examples of how the medication you have been prescribed has helped other patients.

When your doctor is going to prescribe medication for you, it is essential to let them know about any medications you are already taking, such as herbal medicines, over the counter medicines and vitamin supplements that you take. You should also make them aware of your usage of drugs or alcohol, especially if they are excessive.

This is because some of them may be contraindicated for use at the same time as the medicine you are going to be prescribed. A good example is the use of St. John's Wort, which is a natural remedy for depression, for this can have adverse effects if taken at the same time as certain types of anti-depressants.

If you are worried about side effects and want to be able to report them effectively to your doctor, then perhaps keep a pen and paper handy or a dictaphone so that you can note what you are experiencing and give feedback to your doctor. Never rule out the possibility that you could be over-medicated. Some patients who are on too much medication can end up like walking zombies, barely able to function.

If you tend to suffer from allergic reactions and have been prescribed a medication that you have never taken before, then ensure that the first time you take it you are either at the doctor's surgery or have somebody with you in case you develop an adverse reaction to the drug.

If you have a regular prescription for your medication then you might find it helpful to speak to your pharmacist to see whether they offer a repeat prescription service. This usually means that they can automatically collect your prescription from the doctor's surgery for you and dispense it, ready for you to come in to collect when you need it. This can save you lots of time and hassle, but you should still ensure that you visit the doctor regularly for medication reviews. As well, ask your pharmacist about all the side effects of your medication.

It is also your own responsibility to ensure that you take any medication as directed. If you are confused about the instructions given or are not sure about when or how to take your medication then you should check with your doctor or the pharmacist. Information is the key to safety when you are taking medication. Be extra careful when taking several medicines for a mixture of medications could be causing more harm than good. If you have any concerns, speak to your doctor or pharmacist.

You might need to take medication at a certain time of day, or leave a particular amount of time between doses, so it is essential that you adhere to this as you may risk taking too much which could be harmful.

It is also important not to discontinue medication too soon. Antibiotics are a good example of this, even if you are starting to feel better, then you should still continue taking the medicine until you have completed the course, otherwise you run the risk of your infection not being fully treated.

Patients not taking their medication is an increasing burden to the NHS as the prescribed drugs are effectively being wasted and the condition that the patient is suffering from may be worsening, which will lead to the need for more resources to be used for the patient as a result.

Side effects

No matter what sort of medication you need to take there is always a chance that you will experience some sort of side effects. Some people do not experience any at all, whereas others may experience quite significant side effects. The likelihood of your experiencing them can be affected by a number of different factors including your overall health, your age, your gender and how much you weigh. Sometimes, even your ethnicity can affect the way your body reacts to a drug, as can the severity of your medical condition.

You should ensure that you have read the literature that came with the medication and make yourself familiar with the potential side effects that could occur as a result of your medication and be aware of what you need to do if you experience side effects.

No matter how minor the effects that you experience, it is always a good idea to mention them to your doctor. This is because they can be a warning sign or an indication that the medication is not working properly for you. Don't stop taking the medication without discussing it with your doctor, as some drugs can cause a withdrawal reaction if you stop taking them suddenly, so you really need to be aware of the likely effects of stopping.

Unfortunately not all doctors are fully up to speed in medication side effects and how to deal with them, so if you are not happy with what your doctor is telling you, then you should exercise your right as a patient to get a second opinion.

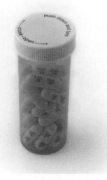

Additionally, if you are going to discuss your medication or any side effects with your doctor, then it is a good idea to research the drug and its effects for yourself. There is an enormous amount of information available on the Internet, but you should always note the source and be aware that not all Internet sources are reputable and/or accurate.

Expiry dates
It may seem strange to think of medication having an expiry date, but if you examine the packaging you will find that most prescription and over the counter drugs do have them.

The expiry date indicates the time period within which the medication will maintain its labelled strength when it is stored in the recommended manner. The expiry date is normally shown as month and year, and should be taken to refer to the last day of the stated month.

The expiry date should be visible on the inner and outer packaging. Some drugs have fairly long expiry dates, whereas others, such as eye drops for example, have a much shorter shelf life. This is because of the possibility of microbial contamination of the liquid.

The problem with using medication after the expiry date has passed is that the strength of the drug may have deteriorated. Unfortunately the answer is not simply to take more of the medicine. This would not be safe because it is not possible to establish what the actual strength of the drug would be at the time.

Another more unusual occurrence is that the drug actually changes its composition over time. This could be potentially very serious and could lead to dangerous side effects so, again, it is absolutely essential that you don't take the risk of ingesting a changed drug by taking it after its expiry date.

Even if the medicine you have is within its expiry date, then you should check that it has been stored according to the manufacturer's instructions. If it hasn't then it could have had an effect on the expiry of the medicine.

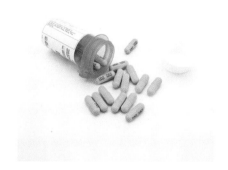

Before drugs are put on the market, stability tests are carried out on them within the containers and packaging that they are being sold in. One of the main causes of drug degradation is the fact that many substances react with atmospheric oxygen. Temperature is another contributing factor.

The actual changes to the medicinal compound that can occur include changes in pH level, particle sizes can alter and the dissolution rate of tablets or capsules can be affected. Changes in pH level are particularly worrying as they can cause serious tissue damage.

Contraindications

A contraindication is something that makes the administration of a particular medicine or the implementation of a particular medical procedure inadvisable because the associated risks are heightened.

A good example is when someone has experienced a previous allergic reaction to a drug. This is very common with penicillin and patients who have previously developed an allergic reaction to penicillin should not take it again in future.

Some contraindications are total, usually referred to as absolute, meaning that there are no circumstances in which the drug or procedure should be given. Others can be considered as relative, which means that there are considerable risks, but that they can be weighed up against the benefits and that they can b managed appropriately.

Contraindications can also mean that you should not use certain products whilst taking a certain type of medication. Other drugs, types of personal care products and varieties of food may have to be avoided whilst taking a course of medication.

Pharmacists

It takes five years to become qualified as a pharmacist. They take a 4-year degree followed by a year of 'hands on' experience. After this they can then register with the Royal Pharmaceutical Society of Great Britain.

Pharmacists offer several health services that you may not be aware of and that may save you having to make an appointment with your doctor. Pharmacists in the UK are estimated to undertake around 57 million consultations every year.

They can offer advice on the safe use of medicines, both over the counter and prescription. They can usually offer a Medicines Use review which is a detailed chat in private about your medication.

If you have a minor illness or ailment then it is worth going to see your local pharmacist as they are likely to be able to offer advice and recommendations for treatment.

Some pharmacies operate specific minor ailment services which means that the pharmacist can assess and advise you, recommend medicines and even issue prescriptions in some circumstances. They will not hesitate to refer you to your GP if they believe it is necessary.

Conditions that your pharmacist will be able to advise you on include:

Eczema.
Acne.
Coughs.
Colds.
Cuts and bruises.
Constipation.
Allergies.
Aches and pains.
Indigestion.
Diarrhoea.
Threadworms.
Period pain.
Thrush.
Warts.
Verrucas.
Mouth ulcers.
Cold sores.
Athlete's foot.
Nappy rash.
Teething.

If you need emergency contraception you can go to the pharmacist who will be able to provide the morning-after pill over the counter after a brief consultation.

Pregnancy testing is commonly available in pharmacies.

If you are a user of needles and syringes then they will be able to offer an exchange service to you. Pharmacists can also dispose of unused medicines safely.

The pharmaceutical industry

Don't forget that the drug companies are extremely powerful and place a lot of pressure on doctors to prescribe their products. The more cynical would say that the medical profession has been 'sold' to the pharmaceutical industry.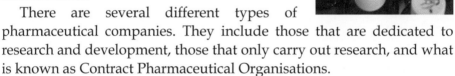

The pharmaceutical industry in the UK is the second largest contributor to GDP. The biggest pharmaceutical companies in the UK are GlaxoWelcome, SmithKlineBeecham and Astra Zeneca.

There are several different types of pharmaceutical companies. They include those that are dedicated to research and development, those that only carry out research, and what is known as Contract Pharmaceutical Organisations.

These CPOs operate field sales teams, both dedicated and syndicated.

Dedicated sales teams work with one particular company to promote a single drug over a sustained period of time. Syndicated sales teams sell up to three different drugs at any one time.

There are several different types of drug company sales representatives:

Part Time Medical Representative
They normally work in the morning, making visits to Primary Care customers.

Full Time Medical Representative
They make visits to Primary Care customers such as GPs, practice nurses and practice managers. Sometimes they visit Health Authorities.

Full Time GP/Hospital Representative
Their time is split between visits to GPs and hospitals.

Hospital Specialist
They are experienced representatives who have worked within Primary Care and can then specialise 100% in hospital visits.

Specialist PCG Representatives

These representatives are employed to work directly with Primary Care Groups to influence their decision-making.

The power and wealth of the drug companies is absolutely staggering. According to IMS Health, which produces statistics relating to the pharmaceutical industry, worldwide drug sales are worth around $400 billion dollars every year. It is estimated that the world's five largest drug companies are together worth more than twice the GNP of all the countries of sub-Saharan Africa.

This level of wealth gives the pharmaceutical companies immense influence politically which is obviously a desirable state of affairs for them. In order to try and maintain this level of power and influence, it is essential that the drug companies find ways of maintaining the steady flow of cash, one of which is the constant increase in drug prices and the other being to promote their products directly to the doctors who write prescriptions for their patients.

Many drug company representatives give gifts or organise hospitality for doctors. Even though most countries have in place guidelines and codes of conduct for pharmaceutical companies, when it comes to marketing their products, many manage to circumvent the guidelines in order to use their persuasive techniques on doctors and market their products. It is said that the pharmaceutical industry spends around twice the amount on marketing as it does on research and development.

In a quite recent case, Schering-Plough were found to be paying large amounts of money to doctors in the form of 'consulting fees' and doctors were also paid to conduct so-called 'clinical trials' which would involve them prescribing a particular drug for a period of several months and being paid by the drug company.

Some companies also run Continuing Medical Education courses, which usually involve trips to exotic destinations and being wined and dined throughout. Whilst the courses are supposed to be informing medical professionals about a certain condition, they all too often take the format of an advertising exercise, with a particular product being promoted as an effective treatment with no reference to other alternatives.

The *New York Times* recently reported that in the US, approximately half of the CME courses, which take place every year, are sponsored

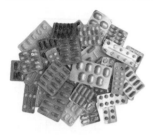

by the pharmaceutical industry. This raises serious questions about the possible bias that is present and the potential influencing of doctors who prescribe medication to patients.

In the UK, there is only one major purchaser, the NHS. This is known as a 'monopolist market' which begs the question as to the need for there to be so much focus on sales.

The NHS is divided into two sectors – Primary and Secondary Care. Primary Care relates to general practice, whereas Secondary Care relates to hospital care. Although the two sectors work very much in conjunction with one another, ten times more prescribing takes place in the Primary Care section.

Doctors in the Primary Care sector work from a prescribing guide, issued by the Primary Care Group. Drugs included within this guide are more likely to be prescribed to patients than those that are not.

The main source of income for a pharmaceutical company is an in-patient prescription drug. The gross margin on these products is very high. Other products offered by pharmaceutical companies include generic drugs and over the counter drugs.

Generic drugs are not as profitable because other companies can produce them so there is competition which drives down prices and profit margins. Over the counter drugs, which are sometimes referred to as 'ethical' drugs for some reason, are very much a consumer product and as such are less profitable. There is usually a lot of focus on marketing this type of product.

A successfully patented drug can generate up to £1 million pounds a day in revenue for the pharmaceutical company behind it. Once the patent expires, however, then the drug can be manufactured by other companies under its generic name, which can then be sold much more cheaply, so the original company then has to develop new drugs with patents to get their revenue back up again.

Drug company sales representatives usually only promote prescription medications. They carry out sales visits to doctors to encourage them to prescribe their drug, and their sales results are determined by the number of prescriptions dispensed by pharmacists.

In the case of vaccines, these are not dependent on the doctor choosing to prescribe them but are usually purchased by the doctor directly from the pharmaceutical company.

Strangely, the representatives do not usually sell directly to the pharmacist. They simply order the drugs that doctors have been prescribing from their wholesaler.

(Source: Gordan, 2002)

Procedures
A medical procedure can be defined as the act of diagnosis, treatment or operation.

Procedures can be grouped into:

> Propedeutic Procedures.
> Diagnostic Procedures.
> Theraputic Procedures.
> Surgical Procedures.

Propedeutic procedures
Propedeutic means 'introductory instruction' and these types of procedure are simple checks that a doctor uses to help him check your health.

Medical inspections
This means a basic observational check of your skin, ears, eyes, weight, respiration, odour, muscle tone, hair and movement.

Palpation
Palpation means to touch or manipulate, so this sort of examination is when the doctor physically touches the body to check for lumps or assess where there might be pain or inflammation.

Percussion

When examining the chest or abdomen the doctor will firmly tap the skin at regular intervals which helps them to establish what is below the surface.

Auscultation

This is the term for when the doctor uses an instrument such as a stethoscope to listen to the sounds inside the body.

Temperature

Diagnostic procedures

This refers to the process of attempting to determine and identify a possible disease or disorder and the opinion reached by this process.

Amniocentesis

This is a test carried out during pregnancy to determine whether the baby has a serious abnormality.

Barium enema

This is a special type of X-ray which enables a clear image to be generated of the large bowel.

Biopsy

This is a medical procedure which takes a small sample of tissue so that it can be analysed for the presence of abnormal cells.

Cardiac stress test

This test reflects (indirectly) arterial blood flow to the heart during physical exercise. This is then compared to the flow when the patient is at rest, which can then show any imbalances of blood flow to the heart.

Cervical screening

This is the scraping of cells from the cervix in order to detect abnormalities.

Chloride test

This is used to detect pH imbalances and also known as a CI Test.

Electrocardiography
This is the electronic monitoring of the heart.

Electroencephalography
Also known as EEG, this is a method of recording the electrical activity taking place in the brain.

Endoluminal capsule monitoring
A tiny wireless radio transmitter is embedded into a watertight capsule which the patient swallows. Information can be gathered as the capsule makes its way through the digestive system.

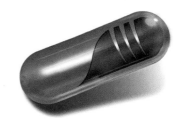

Electrocorticography
This is a procedure which involves placing electrodes onto the exposed surface of the brain during surgery to monitor activity in the cerebral cortex.

Electromyography
This is an electronic method of monitoring muscle activity.

Electronystagmography
This is a test to record involuntary movements of the eye.

Electroculography
This procedure measures the resting potential of the retina.

Electroretinography
This is a measurement of the electrical responses in the retina.

Evoked potential
This is a test which measures the amount of time it takes nerves to respond to a stimulus.

Endoscopy

This is the general name given to the type of procedures that involve using an endoscope to examine the inside of your body. An endoscope is a long, thin, flexible tube which contains a light and a tiny camera so that the doctor can see inside the part of the body that requires examination.

These are the most common procedures of this type:

Colonoscopy – Colon.
Gastroscopy – Oesophagus, stomach and duodenum.
Cystoscopy - Bladder.
Sigmoidoscopy – Rectum and lower part of the bowel.
Colposcopy – Cervix, vagina and vulva.
Otoscopy - Ear.
Ophthalmoscopy - Eye.
Laparoscopy - Abdomen.

Medical imaging

There is a wide variety of medical imaging procedures which can assist with diagnosis by producing images of the inside of the body.

Angiography

This technique uses a special dye to make the blood vessels more visible.

Cerebral angiography - Brain.
Coronary angiography – Heart arteries.
Renal angiography - Kidney.
Pulmonary angiography - Lungs.
Lymph angiography – Lymphatic system.
Retinal angiography – Eye.

Magnetic resonance imaging

Magnetic Resonance Imaging is a medical imaging procedure also referred to as an MRI scan. It uses a magnetic field in conjunction with radio waves to produce pictures of the inside

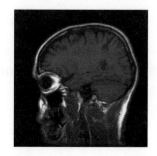

of your body. They are often used for examination of the brain, spine, abdomen and pelvis.

Computerised tomography

Computerised tomography is more commonly known as a CT Scan. It is a painless procedure that uses X-rays to produce very detailed images of the inside of your body.

Positron emission tomography

Also known as a PET Scan, Positron Emission Tomography detects a radioactive substance which is deliberately introduced into the body, which then enables a three-dimensional colour image of the inside of your body to be produced.

Ultrasound scan

This procedure uses high frequency sound waves to create an image from inside the body. It is commonly used during pregnancy to see images of the unborn baby. Ultrasound is also used to examine the heart for signs of enlargement or disease and the prostate gland for cancer.

Therapeutic procedures

A therapeutic effect is a consequence of a medical treatment of any kind, the results of which are judged to be desirable and beneficial. This is true whether the result was expected, unexpected, or even an unintended consequence of the treatment. An adverse effect, on the other hand, is a harmful and undesired effect.

Chemotherapy

This is a treatment for cancer which uses medication to kill malignant cells. The medication is called cytotoxic, and prevents the cancer cells from growing. Sometimes, but not always, chemotherapy on its own will kill all the cancer cells in the body. Usually chemotherapy is used in conjunction with radiotherapy. The treatment is often given after surgery to remove a tumour.

Radiotherapy
Used to treat some types of cancer, radiotherapy uses controlled doses of radiation – usually in the form of X-rays – to target cancer cells in a particular area.

Physiotherapy
Physiotherapy treatments use manipulation and exercise to combat physical problems caused by illness or injury.

Immunisation
Also referred to as vaccination, most immunisations are administered during childhood in the form of an injection. They protect against diseases such as tetanus, polio, pneumococcal infections, diphtheria, meningitis, HPV and MMR. Adults can be given immunisations as well, the common ones include flu and travel related diseases.

Psychotherapy
This is a talking therapy that can be used to help deal with depression and anxiety. It can be carried out individually or as part of a couple or group. There are several different kinds including cognitive behavioural therapy (CBT), person-centred, humanistic, psychoanalysis, and integrated therapy.

Acupuncture
This is a form of traditional Chinese medicine which involves the insertion of very fine needles into specific points around the body as a way of unblocking the flow of energy.

Hormone replacement therapy
This treatment replaces the hormones that your body is no longer producing because of the menopause.

Stem cell transplant
Stem cells can be found in our bone marrow and also from the umbilical cord of a newborn baby. Stem cells produce red and white blood cells as well as platelets. It can be necessary to undergo this type of transplant

because of conditions that affect the blood such as leukaemia or sickle cell anaemia.

Surgical procedures

Surgery is a medical specialty that uses operative manual and instrumental techniques on a patient to investigate or treat a pathological condition such as disease or injury, to help improve bodily function or appearance and sometimes for religious reasons.

Abortion

This is the medical termination of pregnancy.

Adenoidectomy

This is removal of the adenoids which are small lumps of flesh above the tonsils only present in children.

Aortic valve replacement

This is open-heart surgery during which your circulation is taken over by a heart-lung machine.

Cataract surgery

This is the surgical removal of cloudy patches in the lens of the eye.

Circumcision

This is the surgical removal of the foreskin for medical or religious reasons.

Colostomy

A section of the colon is diverted and attached to an external pouch which is used to collect bodily waste.

Cornea transplant

This is the removal of a damaged cornea and replacement with a healthy one from a suitable donor.

Coronary angioplasty
This is a surgical procedure which opens up blocked or narrowed arteries.

Endoscopic surgery
This is quite a common form of surgery during which instruments are passed into the upper gastrointestinal tract to treat problems such as stomach bleeding, varicose veins and swallowing difficulties.

Hand tendon surgery
This operation is carried out when there has been damage to the tendons in your hand.

Laparoscopic surgery
This is a surgical procedure used by doctors to look inside the abdomen. A small incision is made and a laparoscope is then introduced. This is a small thin bendy microscope with a light on the end. The images being picked up can be displayed on a monitor for the surgeon to see what is happening.

Knee replacement therapy
Also known as arthroplasty, this is when a damaged or worn knee joint is replaced with an artificial one which is designed to last for 10 to 15 years.

Your rights when it comes to tests and procedures
If you need to undergo any medical tests then you should ensure that you are fully informed about the results and what the implications are.

If you are advised that you need to undergo a medical procedure then check that it is absolutely necessary. People die because they have undergone unnecessary surgery.

Be aware of what procedures might be available to you. Some doctors will not advise on certain courses of treatment because of their moral or religious beliefs, and sometimes because they feel that the patient has somehow contributed to their own condition and 'don't deserve' the treatment.

If you suspect any of these to be the case and you are informed as to the treatments available then you can ask to see another doctor who will help you. Always remember that you can check the NICE guidelines for the NHS recommended treatments for your condition as a starting point.

Every human being is the author of his own health or disease.

Buddha

Six:
Patients

A patient can be defined as anyone who is on the receiving end of medical treatment, attention or care. This is usually because they are ill or suffering from some sort of injury, although the term 'patient' can refer to someone who is simply visiting a healthcare professional for a routine check-up or examination.

The word originated from a term meaning 'one who suffers'. In some settings you might hear patients being referred to as heath consumers, healthcare consumers, or clients.

Patients can be subdivided into two categories:

Outpatients.
Inpatients.

Outpatients
This type of patient is not kept in hospital overnight, but just visits a clinic or hospital for assessment, diagnosis or treatment. With advances in medical technology, it is even possible to have some types of minor surgery as an outpatient. This is good for the patient and for the NHS because it reduces the pressure on resources and staff which helps to keep the hospital or clinic running smoothly. Normally, only healthy patients can be treated as outpatients in this way.

The care provided to outpatients is sometimes referred to as 'ambulatory care' because of the fact that the procedures performed on an outpatient basis are usually quick and uncomplicated, meaning that patients can literally walk in and out again.

The sort of procedures that can be carried out on outpatients can be for anything from a simple consultation to a psychological therapy session, or even a radiation or chemotherapy treatment for a cancer patient.

Most patients like to attend hospital as an outpatient because it means much less waiting around for them and any recovery can take place in the comfort of their own home. It also means that you don't have to take as much time off from work or other commitments because no hospital stay is required.

Not all procedures can be performed on an outpatient basis. Outpatient appointments on the NHS are usually provided to the patient via the Choose and Book system. This is an electronic system which enables patients to choose the location and time of their appointment.

Inpatients

This type of patient has to stay in hospital for one or more nights. These days, because there have been so many advances in medicine, it is usually only necessary to stay in hospital as an inpatient if you require quite major surgery, or are quite unwell.

It used to be the case that your GP would arrange for you to be admitted to hospital and that they would then visit you on the ward and manage your care. These days, however, most hospitals practise what is known as 'hospitalist care', which is when patients are looked after by doctors who only work at the hospital and specialise in the particular needs of the patients under their care.

Inpatient care dates back to 230 AD, when the very first hospitals were founded in India by Ashoka the Great.

As patients, it can be hard sometimes to keep in mind that we are entitled to a good service from our healthcare providers. All too often we are rushed in and out of appointments. It can feel like we are on a conveyor belt. Sometimes it feels like medical staff treat us simply as a number and not as a human being at all.

When you see a doctor, give them as much detail as you can. Write down everything that you want to communicate with them as it is easy to forget everything you want to say once in the consultation room. Don't be afraid to question or challenge your doctor. It is your body and you have a right to get the best advice and information.

In years gone by, the relationship between doctor and patient was very distant, almost anonymous, whereas today patients can be much more involved in their own healthcare decisions.

If you are physically and mentally able to, then there is no reason why your relationship with your doctor should not be as equal partners who each have a set of different interests in the relationship.

Until it was abolished in 2001, there was a Patients Charter which set out your rights as a patient and indicated what you could expect from the NHS. This charter was then replaced with a publication from the Department of Health entitled *Your Guide to the NHS: Getting the most from your National Health Service*, which gave an overview of the NHS for patients. The publication is no longer available.

Patient confidentiality

As patients, we have an understandable desire to know that the deeply personal information held within our medical records remains confidential and is protected as much as is humanly possible.

There have been a number of high profile data breaches in recent years. A recent news article reported on the fact that doctors using social networking services such as Facebook and Twitter were breaching patient confidentiality by posting details about patients and cases on the Internet in the course of discussion.

The BBC report detailed figures from research carried out by the journal of the American Medical Association. The statistics showed that out of 78 medical schools in the USA, over half of them had reported incidences of doctors posting content online which violated patient confidentiality. At the present time, the GMC does not have any guidelines which govern the conduct of doctors on the Internet.

The BBC also reported an incident in which medical records were left unattended in a corridor at a Scottish hospital. A member of the public discovered the crates containing the medical records at the Southern General in Glasgow. A BBC reporter was made aware of the issue and visited the location a few days later to see for themselves only to find the records still in the corridor with no obvious security measures.

NHS Greater Glasgow and Clyde admitted that the records should have been stored in sealed boxes and that they should have had a member of staff with them whilst they were waiting to be transferred to a new storage area.

(Source: BBC, 2009)

The NHS is obliged both legally and ethically to maintain the absolute confidentiality of patient records. NHS Caldicott Guardians are senior members of staff from throughout the NHS and Social Services who have been appointed to protect patient information. There are around 750 of them in total. The appointment of the Caldicott Guardians came as a result of a 1997 report (the Caldicott Report) which pinpointed weaknesses in the way that confidential patient information was handled by parts of the NHS.

The guardians have a set of guidelines which are laid out in their manual which is centred around six principles that were identified in the Caldicott Report. These principles are:

Principle 1
Justify the purpose(s) for using confidential information.

Principle 2
Only use it when absolutely necessary.

Principle 3
Use the minimum that is required.

Principle 4
Access should be on a strict need-to-know basis.

Principle 5
Everyone must understand his or her responsibilities.

Principle 6
Understand and comply with the law.

Anything said by you as a patient to your doctor is protected under the Data Protection Act. The knowledge that whatever you tell them is confidential is crucial to the trust that is necessary in a doctor-patient relationship. This premise formed part of the Hippocratic Oath - the basis for modern medical ethics.

There are some very narrow circumstances within which information might be revealed, for example if the non-communication of the information would put others at risk.

Worryingly, however, the GMC is currently considering proposals to make identifiable patient records available to medical researchers. The new proposals will allow records to be given to medical researchers if it is deemed to be in the public interest and that it would be unreasonably difficult to contact the patient in question.

(Source: Edwards, 2009)

Getting advice

As a patient it can often be useful to have a plan of action in place prior to seeing a doctor or other healthcare professional so you can make sure that you find out everything you need to know. In most circumstances, when you have a health issue, the first person that you make contact with is your GP. They can make a first diagnosis and give you some advice on your condition and will also assess whether you need to see a specialist. If you want to have private treatment they will be able to suggest hospitals or contacts and possible costs. Don't feel intimidated by your GP, this is what they are paid to do.

Before your appointment

Before you go to see your GP it is a good idea to make a list of your symptoms. There may also be questions that you want to ask your doctor, so you might want to write these down as well. Examples of questions are:

What is wrong with me?
What tests do I need?
What treatment choices are there?
Are there any risks or side effects to the treatment?

Will I have to go into hospital?
How long will I be in hospital?
How long will the treatment take?
Will I have to take time off work?

During your appointment

Your doctor will ask you to tell them about your symptoms. You should refer to your list to make sure that you don't miss anything out. If the doctor asks you any questions make sure you give truthful and accurate answers as they may affect the treatments that you can be offered. The doctor might want to examine you or carry out some basic health checks.

Once the initial assessment has been made, then the doctor will be able to tell you their opinion on what is wrong with you. It can be useful to take notes while they are explaining things to you as it is easy to forget what has been said once you are outside the consultation room.

If the GP thinks that you need to see a specialist, then they will explain this to you and issue a referral letter.

Seeing a specialist

In many ways, you can follow the same procedure when seeing a specialist that you followed when seeing your GP. You might want to consider asking some different questions such as:

How many of these operations do you do/have you done?
What are your audit results?
Has your audit been published?
What is your failure rate?
What is your wound infection rate?
How do you compare with the national average?

The specialist or consultant will be able to give you lots of information during your appointment, so you may want to take some notes. The information you are given might include:

Whether you need to undergo surgery.
What will happen during the procedure.

How long the procedure will take.
What anaesthetic you will need.
Whether you can be treated as an outpatient or an inpatient.
What sort of pain you can expect.
Whether there will be any scarring.
Whether there are any risks.
Whether you need to follow any special diets or regimes prior to surgery.
How long it will take you to recover.
What aftercare you will need.

Patient choice

NHS patients have the right to make choices about many aspects of their treatment. This is because research has shown that treatments are more effective if patients fully understand them and have been involved in choosing them.

The main choices that you have within the NHS are:

The right to choose a GP.
The right to choose which hospital you go to.
The right to be involved in decisions about your care.

The NHS constitution sets out in more detail exactly what you can expect from the NHS. It came into force in January 2009 and eventually the law will ensure that all parties that work with the NHS have to adhere to the principles within it. There are plans to review the constitution every 10 years.

The main rights that are set out for you, the patient, are as follows:

Access to healthcare

The right to free NHS treatment.
The right to access NHS services.
The right to expect that local needs will be served by the NHS.
The right to go to other EU countries for treatment if necessary.
The right not to be discriminated against on the basis of gender, race, religion, sexual orientation or disability.

Quality of care and environment

The right to a professional standard of care.

The right to expect that the NHS will monitor and improve their performance.

Nationally approved drugs, treatments and programmes

The right to drugs and treatments approved by NICE.

The right to expect local treatment decisions to be made rationally.

The right to receive vaccinations.

Respect, consent and confidentiality

The right to be treated with dignity and respect.

The right to accept or refuse treatment.

The right to be given information about your treatment in advance.

The right to privacy and confidentiality.

The right of access to your health records.

Informed choice

The right to choose your GP practice.

The right to prefer a particular doctor.

The right to make choices about your care.

Involvement in your healthcare and in the NHS

The right to be involved in discussions and decisions about your healthcare.

The right to be involved in the planning of healthcare services.

Complaint and redress

The right to have any complaint dealt with.

The right to know the outcome of any investigation.

The right to take your complaint to the Ombudsman.

The right to make a claim for judicial review.

The right to compensation where you have been harmed by negligent treatment.

Patient responsibilities

The NHS constitution also sets out some guidelines for our responsibilities as patients. These are designed to ensure that resources are used effectively and that the NHS can function at an optimal level.

We all have a responsibility for our own health and well-being and must recognise that we can contribute to it significantly. We must ensure that we are registered with a GP, as this is the main method of accessing NHS care.

We should treat NHS staff with respect and not risk prosecution by causing disturbances or nuisance on NHS property. Any information about our health and status should be provided to healthcare workers. Appointments should be kept or cancelled as appropriate. Any treatment prescribed should be followed and completed.

We should participate in public health programmes such as vaccination. We must ensure that close relatives, friends and carers are aware of our wishes regarding organ donation. We should give feedback, whether negative or positive, in respect of the care we have received.

Doctor-patient boundaries

The doctor-patient relationship is completely based on trust. The patient must be able to trust their doctor in order to be able to discuss personal medical matters with them.

Doctors have a responsibility to behave in a certain way with their patients so as to facilitate this trust-based relationship. The core guidance produced by the GMC for doctors, Good Medical Practice, sets out three basic principles, which are:

You must not use your professional position to establish or pursue a sexual or improper emotional relationship with a patient or someone close to them.

You must treat patients with dignity.

You must protect patients from the risk of harm posed by another colleague's conduct. The safety of patients must come first at all times. If you have concerns that a colleague may not be fit to practise, you must take appropriate steps without delay, so that the concerns are investigated and patients protected where necessary.

When you are having a consultation with your doctor it is important to feel that these principles are being adhered to. If they are not, and the doctor-patient boundary is being breached, then it can undermine your trust in the doctor as well as that of the general public in the medical profession.

It is always important to keep in mind that there is an imbalance of power between doctor and patient due to the amount of specialist knowledge and professional skills that the doctor possesses, as against the patient needing their help and advice and perhaps being in a position of vulnerability because of emotional or mental considerations.

Sexual and emotional relationships

Doctors should not attempt to pursue a sexual relationship with you as a patient or someone close to you. If you have been a patient of theirs in the past, but are not any longer, it is still inappropriate for them to pursue a relationship with you if you were vulnerable because of your age or state of mental health at the time of consulting them. By the same token, if your former doctor – no matter how long ago it was – tries to start a relationship with you, it may still be seen as an abuse of their professional relationship with you.

Intimate examinations

None of us particularly enjoy having medical examinations, especially if they are of an intimate nature. If you wish then you are perfectly entitled to ask for a chaperone to be present with you who can be a friend or relative, or perhaps another staff member. If it is not possible for your chaperone to be present then you can ask for the examination to be carried out at another time when they can be with you.

If your doctor tells you that you need to have an intimate examination then they should explain to you exactly why it is necessary. They should also tell you what the examination will entail and whether it will be painful or uncomfortable. If you want to ask questions then you are entitled to do so. They should obtain your permission prior to carrying out the examination – you do not have to give permission for the examination to go ahead if you don't want to.

The doctor should give you some privacy if you need to get undressed. They should not assist you with removing your clothing unless you have asked them to.

During the examination the doctor should tell you what they are doing and should stop if you ask them to. They should not make any personal comments during the examination.

Inappropriate behaviour

A doctor should behave appropriately with you at all times. They should not use acts, words or behaviour of a sexual nature at any time during your consultation with them.

Personal beliefs

Our beliefs and values are central to all of our lives and this is also true of doctors. It is important to be aware that some doctors may have personal beliefs which could affect the advice and treatment that they offer you. Their first duty should be, however, to offer you the best care possible. You have a right to complain if you feel that a doctor is discriminating against you because of your:

Age.
Culture.
Colour.
Disability.
Ethnicity.
Gender.
Lifestyle.
Status.
Race.
Religion.
Sexual orientation.

You are also entitled not to be subjected to any discussion on personal beliefs by the doctor. They should not try to impose their views on you or make inappropriate comments about your personal beliefs or circumstances. If you require assistance with treatment or procedures that the doctor has a conscientious objection to, such as abortion, then you are entitled to see another doctor who can advise you appropriately.

If you have any concerns about the conduct of a doctor then you are entitled to make a complaint against them. You would usually make a complaint in the first instance at the place where you have been treated by the doctor in question. If you are in England, this will be via the complaints procedure of the NHS or Primary Care trust; in Scotland to your local board of NHS Scotland; in Wales to your local Health Board or NHS trust, and in Northern Ireland to your Health and Social Care Board or the Patient and Client Council.

If the doctor that you wish to complain about is working in the private sector, then you should approach the private hospital or clinic that they work for, or the Citizens Advice Bureau.

In very serious cases you can make a complaint directly to the General Medical Council. A serious case would be classed as:

> Making mistakes in diagnosis or treatment.
> Failure to examine a patient properly.
> Fraud or dishonesty.
> Confidentiality breaches.
> Criminal offences.

The GMC would then undertake an investigation as required.

In health there is freedom.
Health is the first of all liberties.

Henri Frederic Amiel

Seven:
Children's Health

Children have a unique set of health needs which as parents we have a duty to recognise. The Healthy Child Programme is the framework of review, vaccinations, screening and tests that takes place whilst your child is growing up. In each geographical area, there is a Healthy Child team led by health visitors who work alongside GPs and Sure Start staff to facilitate the programme for your child.

When your baby is born you will be given a 'red book' or Personal Child Health Record in which your child's progress will be recorded as they are growing up. Every time you have contact with any healthcare professionals regarding your child the visit will be recorded in the 'red book' alongside details of vaccinations, screening and tests. Take it with you whenever your child has to attend hospital or see the GP and fill in the developmental questionnaires.

Babies

If you are a parent for the first time, then caring for a baby can be a daunting experience. Babies' needs are fairly simple, they need to be fed, kept clean and warm and given love.

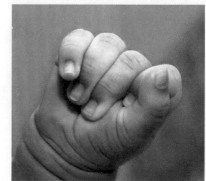

Babies will be given developmental reviews by the health visitor at certain milestones:

14 days.
6 to 8 weeks.
3 months.
4 months.
1 year.

There are a series of screening tests that will take place during their life which start at birth with:

Newborn hearing test to check whether hearing is normal.
Newborn physical examination when heart, hips, and eyes are all checked.
Newborn bloodspot test for phenylketonuria, congenital hypothyroidism, cystic fibrosis and sickle cell disorders.

Obviously babies cannot tell you if they are ill, so you need to be aware of any signs and symptoms they have. Common conditions in babies include:

Bronchiolitis
This is a respiratory infection that affects babies. Symptoms are similar to a cold but go on for longer. Some babies with this condition need to have oxygen, so take your baby to the doctor or hospital if you suspect they might have it. Take them immediately if:

They are coughing a lot.
They are very breathless.
They are more sleepy than usual.
They are not feeding well.
They are wheezing.
Their skin is changing colour.

Febrile convulsions

These are fits which can occur in babies who have a high temperature. It is frightening to experience but it will soon pass. The signs that a fit is occurring are:

Loss of consciousness.
Stiff or floppy limbs.
Stopping breathing for up to 30 seconds.
Twitching limbs.
Rolling eyes.
Soiling or wetting their nappy during the convulsion.

If they are experiencing a fit for the first time then you should take them to Accident and Emergency. If they have had one before then contact NHS Direct or your GP. Call an ambulance if:

The convulsion goes on for more than 5 minutes.
There is no improvement in your child's condition when the fit has ended.
Your child has breathing difficulties.
Another convulsion starts.

Meningitis

This is a serious condition that in its bacterial form can be life-threatening. If you suspect meningitis, then you should take your child to Accident and Emergency immediately as time is of the essence when treating meningitis. The symptoms can include:

Raised Temperature.
Vomiting.
High pitched crying.
Blank expression.
Pale complexion.
Floppiness.
Not wanting to be handled.
Neck retraction and back arching.

Convulsions.

Lethargy.

Bulging soft spot.

Rash of red or purple spots that does not fade when you press a glass against it.

Anaphylactic shock

This is a severe allergic reaction that affects the whole body and can be life-threatening. If you suspect it has occurred to your child call an ambulance immediately. The signs are:

Breathing difficulties.

Facial swelling.

Swallowing problems.

A blotchy rash.

Fainting.

Nausea and vomiting.

Vomiting and diarrhoea

Very common in children, they are easily caught by little babies. It is important to try and keep giving fluids so as to avoid dehydration. Take your baby to the doctor if:

The symptoms last for more than 24 hours.

They have signs of dehydration - no wet nappies, sunken soft spot.

Children aged 1 to 5

Children will continue to be monitored by the health visitor with a review at:

2 years old.

School entry.

Reviews will cover:

General development.

Growth.

Healthy eating.
Keeping active.
Dental care.
Behaviour.
Sleeping habits.
Safety.
Vaccinations.
Weight.
Height.
Hearing.
Vision.

This age group is still building up immunity to the many illnesses that are present in our society so there are several things that you can expect.

Colds
Colds are very common for this age group, they can catch as many as eight in a year. They should get better in a week and do not require treatment with antibiotics.

Ear infections
These can go hand in hand with a cold and may cause a high temperature. They are not usually treated with antibiotics. If it has affected your child's hearing for more than two to six weeks you should take them to the doctor.

Glue ear
This develops as a result of repeated middle ear infections and can be made worse if parents smoke. Sticky fluids build up and can affect hearing so you should see your child's GP.

Sore throats
These are usually caused by colds and clear up quite quickly. See your GP if it continues for more than four days or causes difficulty swallowing.

Coughs

Often present at the same time as a cold, most coughs are nothing to worry about. If it continues for a long time then you should see your GP.

Chickenpox

The symptoms include a rash of itchy blisters, temperature and general lethargy. Take your child to the doctor who will probably give them paracetamol or ibuprofen to relieve their temperature and calamine lotion to soothe any itching.

Measles

Quite rare these days because of the MMR vaccine, measles can become serious. It starts like a cold with watery eyes and a rash appearing around about the fourth day. Take your child to the GP if they are having trouble breathing, are coughing a lot or seem drowsy.

Mumps

Also rare because of the MMR vaccine, mumps can be distinguished by a swelling around the face. There is no need to see the doctor unless they develop a stomach ache or develop a rash.

Parvovirus B19 (also known as fifth disease or slapped cheek disease)

So called because of the bright red mark that appears on the cheeks, you only need to seek medical advice if your child suffers from other health problems.

Rubella

German measles or rubella can be difficult to diagnose. It begins like a cold, and then flat spots develop. Anyone with rubella should stay away from pregnant women.

Whooping cough

This is similar to a cold and cough, but the cough gets worse. After about two weeks, coughing bouts commence which can make it difficult to breathe. The condition can last up to three months and is so called because a 'whooping' noise accompanies the coughing. See your GP if you suspect whooping cough.

Whilst it is true that young children of this age group pick up minor illnesses very frequently, it doesn't mean that they never become seriously ill. If you suspect that your child is suffering from meningitis or another serious condition then you must take them to Accident and Emergency.

Most doctors are happy to be safe rather than sorry, so don't feel like you will be wasting their time if it turns out to be nothing. Conversely, if you feel that the doctor is not taking your concerns seriously, then be assertive and stand up for your right to get a second opinion.

Children aged 6 to 15

An enormous amount of growth takes place during this time with many milestones in your child's development being passed. Whilst general health concerns will not be very different from those that have come before, older children have more stress and pressure to deal with as they go through the school system. This can lead to mental health issues such as depression which you sh uld be aware of.

This is also a time for ensuring that healthy diet and exercise play a part in your child's life with a gradual emphasis on helping them to make healthy choices for themselves. You can start to educate them about cooking and eating healthily and encourage them to engage in physical activity.

Older children and teenagers will need to be educated about puberty, sex and contraception.

Vaccinations

In the UK there is an ongoing programme of vaccinations for children. Children are invited for vaccination at certain times during their life, and all vaccinations are free of charge.

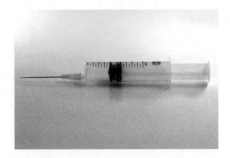

Vaccinations work by introducing a tiny amount of a particular bacterium or virus into the body in order to encourage the immune system to produce antibodies and memory cells. If the body is exposed to the bacterium in the future, the memory cells will activate and protect the person against the illness.

Many serious illnesses around the world have been eradicated because of vaccination so it is seen as important to maintain vaccination programmes to ensure that illnesses do not reappear in the future.

There are often concerns reported in the press about the safety of vaccines, however they are not licensed without extensive safety testing. The effectiveness of vaccines is then monitored on an ongoing basis to ensure that they remain safe.

After being vaccinated, some babies and children might feel a little bit unwell, but this should pass quickly and they can be given paracetamol or ibuprofen to relieve any symptoms. If your baby or child is ill with a temperature then you should not take them to be vaccinated. Make a new appointment for them when they are better.

Starting at two months they will have:

Diphtheria.
Tetanus.
Whooping cough.
Polio.
HiB.

These are then repeated at three months and four months. A HiB booster is given at 12 months.

The Pneumococcal Conjugate vaccine (PCV) protects against meningitis, severe ear infections and pneumonia. It is administered at two months, four months and 13 months.

MenC, which protects against meningitis and septicaemia, is given at three, four and 12 months.

The MMR (measles, mumps & rubella) vaccine is given at 13 months and three years four months.

Girls aged between 12 and 13 are given the HPV, and girls and boys between 13 and 18 are given Td and IPV.

There are other vaccinations which may or may not be offered depending on the policy in your area.

In some cases the tuberculosis BCG is given at birth. This can be given if it is thought that the baby might come into contact with TB and would be at risk if they were not vaccinated.

Hepatitis B is also sometimes given at birth. This is usually because the mother tests positive for Hepatitis B or has had acute Hepatitis B during pregnancy.

If you are going to be travelling abroad with your child, and are going to be travelling to certain areas, you may be required to have them vaccinated against certain conditions. This may be a condition of your entering that country.

Whilst vaccinations are highly recommended, you are not required by law to have your child vaccinated. It is your decision and you should feel free to decide for yourself whether to have your child vaccinated.

Some children should not be vaccinated with live vaccines if they are being treated for a serious condition such as cancer, or are immunosuppressed. Anyone who has previously suffered from an allergic reaction to the vaccine should not be given it again. If in doubt, tell the healthcare professional who is going to carry out the vaccination so that they can assess whether it should be given or not.

Accidents

For children over the age of one, accidental injury is one of the biggest causes of child death in the UK, killing more children than illnesses such as leukaemia and meningitis. Many accidents could be avoided by taking some basic safety precautions.

Most accidents happen in the home so it is important to ensure that your home is as safe as possible. The living room, kitchen, stairs and bedroom are the most common places for children to have an accident at home. If your child is hurt then you should take them to hospital if they:

Have lost consciousness.
Have stopped breathing.

Are vomiting.

Are drowsy.

Have swallowed something they shouldn't have.

Are bleeding from the ears.

Are bleeding heavily.

May have internal injuries.

Are complaining of severe pain.

Safety measures that you can take at home include:

Fitting window restrictors.

Fitting stair gates.

Keeping balcony doors locked.

Making sure furniture is secured to the wall so it cannot be pulled over.

Keeping small objects away from children.

Having an awareness of cords or ribbons on clothing.

Laying babies on their back to sleep.

Keeping plastic bags away from children.

Fitting smoke alarms.

Taking care to switch off heated appliances.

Keeping hot drinks away from children.

Keeping young children out of the kitchen.

Making sure bath water is not too hot.

Keeping anything poisonous locked away.

Disposing of old medicines.

Not leaving children unsupervised in the bath or a paddling pool.

Children in hospital

It can be very daunting for a child to have to go into hospital, but there are things that you can do to make it less frightening for them. There are lots of story books available that are about going into hospital which you can read with them and you could also use their dolls or teddies to play doctors and nurses.

You should practise these activities with all children as they are likely to have to attend hospital at some stage and it is better for them to be prepared and knowledgeable about what to expect.

Even if your child is very little, you should still explain everything that is happening to them and be truthful about things such as pain. If possible you should stay with them as much as you can in the hospital, as this will be reassuring for them. Most hospitals have facilities for parents to stay with their children overnight.

Let hospital staff know about any special words your child uses and take their favourite comforter or cuddly toy into the hospital with them.

Special needs

Some children are born with or develop serious conditions or have special needs. In these situations your family needs as much help and support as you can get to help you deal with the situation.

You will probably have to have a lot of contact with your GP, and you should feel confident about asking questions to do with your child's condition. The sort of things that you might want to ask them include:

What is the name of my child's condition?
Do they need to have any medical tests?
Will the condition get worse?
What should I do if they need urgent medical help?
Are there any support groups for families dealing with the same condition?
What can I do to help my child?

When you are seeing your doctor about your child's condition it can be a good idea to make notes as it is easy to forget what has been discussed once you get home. You might also want to ask a friend or relative to attend appointments with you.

Many children with special needs qualify for extra help at school. Talk to your doctor or health visitor to arrange for a statutory assessment to be carried out by the local authority or health board. This will then enable any extra help to be provided for your child.

Many areas have dedicated child development centres which are there to help children with special needs and their families. They are usually staffed by a team of doctors, therapists, health visitors and social workers and can be a great source of support. Ask your doctor or health visitor if they can refer you to one of these teams.

Other organisations that can offer support to children with special needs and their families are:

Contact a Family: *cafamily.org*

Early Support backed by Sure Start: *earlysupport.org.uk*

The first wealth is health.

Ralph Waldo Emerson

Eight:
Healthcare during
Pregnancy

Pregnancy is a time of unique healthcare needs. There are various choices to be made and factors to be taken into account and a whole new team of healthcare staff to deal with. At a time when you might be feeling nervous and apprehensive, it is especially important to understand what your rights and choices are so that you can have a happy and successful outcome to your pregnancy.

Pregnancy is divided into three trimesters each with its own particular needs.

First trimester
This is when most people find out that they are pregnant and see the midwife for the first time. This will be for what is called your 'booking in appointment'. You will also be sent an appointment for your first ultrasound scan.

Some women experience some light bleeding in very early pregnancy. It can be nothing to worry about, but equally could be a sign that something is wrong so it is important to mention it to your midwife.

Second trimester
Things to look out for during this trimester are:

Pain on urination which can be a sign of a bladder infection which is quite common in pregnancy.

You will be sent an appointment for your second scan and at this stage you might be able to find out the sex of your baby, although it is the policy of some hospitals not to tell you the baby's sex, as they have been taken to court for getting the sex wrong.

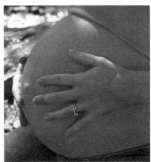

Third trimester
During this trimester you should look out for swelling and high blood pressure as they can be a sign of pre-eclampsia which is a very serious condition.

Seeing your midwife
Going to see your midwife for the first time can be very exciting. You will get to know her quite well over the coming months. There are probably lots of questions you want to ask, so it is a good idea to write a list so you don't forget to ask something when you are having your appointment. Some potential questions are:

> What is my due date?
> What will my antenatal care consist of?
> What tests will I need?
> How do I cope with labour?

At your first appointment you will have some blood taken by the midwife which will be tested for:

> Full blood count.
> Antibodies.
> Blood group and rhesus factor.
> Syphilis.
> Hepatitis B.
> Rubella.
> HIV.

Further blood tests will be taken later on during your pregnancy.

At subsequent appointments she will normally have a feel of your tummy and listen to the baby's heartbeat. You will be asked to take a sample of urine with you each time which will be tested for signs of glucose and protein, which can be indicators of pregnancy diabetes and pre-eclampsia. You will also have your blood pressure taken regularly.

You will normally see the midwife once a month until 28 weeks, then once a fortnight until 36 weeks, and then every week until your baby is born.

Birth options

All pregnant women are entitled to have a choice about where they give birth, although it is of course dependent on the resources available in your local area. Most women tend to give birth in hospital, but there might be a midwife-led birth centre available to you, or you can opt for a home birth.

Your choice of where to give birth will affect what pain relief is available to you. An example of this is that you won't be able to have an epidural if you choose to have a home birth.

Good sources of information about local birth options are:

Children's centres

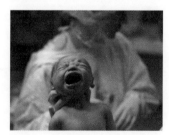

Your GP surgery.
The local maternity unit.
The National Childbirth Trust (NCT).
A supervisor of midwives at your local hospital.

Hospital birth

Reassurance that medical help is close by.
Midwife care.
Doctors on duty.
Various birth choices available.
Full range of pain relief options available.

Home birth
> Familiar surroundings.
> You can be transferred to hospital if necessary.
> Limited pain relief options available.

Midwife-led birth centre
> More relaxed than hospital.
> Lots of support available.
> You can be transferred to hospital if necessary.
> Less choice of pain relief options than in hospital.

Wherever you choose to give birth, you will be encouraged to prepare a birth plan which will set out your wishes and preferences for your labour and birth. It is a good idea to write it down as you may not be able to communicate your wishes effectively whilst in the throes of labour.

Medication during pregnancy

If you need to take any medicine whilst you are pregnant, you must tell the doctor or pharmacist so that they can check that it is safe to do so. Realistically you should avoid as many non-essential medicines as you possibly can. This may mean that you have to cope with minor ailments such as headaches or heartburn without taking anything to ease them.

The decision as to whether you can take a medicine or not can also be affected by what trimester of pregnancy you are in.

First trimester
> Greatest risk period for the baby.
> Internal organs are developing.
> Medicines can affect development.
> Possibility of birth defects.
> Risk of miscarriage.

Second trimester
> Nervous system is developing.
> Medicines can affect birth weight.
> Generally safest period to take any medication.

Third trimester

Medicines can stay in the baby's body after birth.

Can cause breathing difficulties.

Baby may not be able to cope with medicine in bloodstream like mother can.

Throughout the entire pregnancy it is possible that medicines can affect the environment within the womb by causing contractions, decreasing the blood supply or affecting the onset of labour.

Unfortunately it is not possible to be completely certain as to the effect of medicines during pregnancy because it is not possible to carry out clinical trials on pregnant women. The only information that we have is from real life experiences of using medicines over time. This means that very few medicines are licensed for use during pregnancy.

If it is necessary for you to take some medication during pregnancy your doctor will weigh up the potential benefits of the treatment against the possible risks and will make a decision based on those two factors.

There are natural remedies that you can try for minor ailments:

Constipation

Drink more fluid and eat foods that are high in fibre.

Heartburn

Most antacids are safe as long as they don't contain too high a level of sodium.

Pain – headache, backache

Try non-drug methods such as massage or soaking in a warm bath.

Allergies

Reduce your exposure to allergens.

Ask your pharmacist for pregnancy-safe nasal spray and eye drops.

Use steam inhalation.

Colds and coughs

  Drink lots of water.

  Use steam inhalation.

  Suck on lozenges containing honey.

Diarrhoea

  Use rehydration salts.

  Take kaolin mixture.

Eczema

  Use rich moisturisers.

Tests and procedures during pregnancy

Other tests and screening that you might need to have during pregnancy include:

  Ultrasound scans - you will normally have two – a dating scan to check that your baby is growing in line with your expected due date and an anomaly scan which is to check for abnormalities.

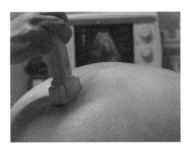

Tests for Down's Syndrome

  Nuchal translucency – this measures the amount of fluid at the back of the baby's neck.

  Combined screening tests – a combination of a scan and blood test.

  Serum screening – blood test.

  Chorionic villus sampling – testing of a sample of the placenta.

  Amniocentesis – testing of a sample of amniotic fluid.

Pain relief during labour

Labour is a painful experience so it is helpful to have some idea of what your pain relief options are going to be. You can write down your preferences in your birth plan so that midwives are clear about your wishes. Some of the techniques available are:

Self help

Learn as much as you can about labour which will make it less frightening.

Use relaxation and breathing techniques to stay calm.

Move around which can really help.

Have a birth partner with you for emotional and practical support during labour.

Have a massage.

Have a bath.

Hydrotherapy

Being in water helps you to relax.

Contractions seem less painful.

Gas and air (also known as entonox)

Reduces the pain.

Makes the pain more bearable.

Is easy to use.

You control it yourself.

Has no harmful side effects.

TENS (Transcutaneous Electrical Nerve Stimulation)

Is effective during active labour.

Can be used in a home birth situation.

Has no side effects.

Injections (pethidine or diamorphine)

Aids relaxation.

Lessens the pain.

Epidural

Is only available in hospital.

Is complete pain relief.

Can only be administered by an anaesthetist.

Natural method

Acupuncture.

Aromatherapy.

Homeopathy.

Hypnosis.

Massage.

Reflexology.

Whatever method of pain relief you choose you should remember that it is your labour and therefore you can make the choice of what you would like to happen. You can deviate from your birth plan, it is only there as a guide. If you change your mind about something, you just need to tell the midwife; just because you started out by saying you don't want an epidural doesn't mean that you can't ask for one later on in labour. Things don't always go to plan so it is important to be open-minded about how you envisage labour to be.

The groundwork of all happiness is health.

Leigh Hunt

Nine:
Private Healthcare
vs
the NHS

Founded in 1948, the NHS is the largest publicly funded health service in the world. It is free at the point of use for the residents of the United Kingdom – over 61 million people.

The organisation employs around 1.5 million people, approximately half of whom are qualified medical professionals of some description.

The NHS deals with one million patients every 36 hours which equates to 463 a minute or eight every second.

The NHS costs over £90 billion a year to run, which is equivalent to a contribution of £1,500 annually by every adult and child in the UK. 60% of the budget goes towards staffing costs.

The NHS has had three core principles since its inception:

It meets the needs of all people.
It is free at the point of delivery.
It is based on clinical need, not the ability to pay.

These core principles were added to in July 2000 as part of a modernisation programme, and now include:

The NHS will provide a comprehensive range of services.

The NHS will shape its services around the needs and preferences of individual patients, their families and carers.

The NHS will respond to the different needs of different populations.

The NHS will work continuously to improve the quality of services and to minimise errors.

The NHS will support and value its staff.

Public funds for healthcare will be devoted solely to NHS patients.

The NHS will work with others to ensure a seamless service for patients.

The NHS will help to keep patients healthy and work to reduce health inequalities.

The NHS will respect the confidentiality of individual patients and provide open access to information about services, treatment and performance.

(Source: NHS, 2009)

NHS structure

The NHS is funded by the Department of Health and is divided into two parts – primary care and secondary care.

Primary care is the frontline of the NHS and incorporates services such as GPs, NHS Direct, walk-in centres, opticians, pharmacists and dentists. Primary Care Trusts (PCTs) are responsible for administering services on a local basis in conjunction with Strategic Health Authorities. PCTs control around 80% of the NHS budget, overseeing 29,000 GPs and 18,000 dentists.

Also known as acute care, secondary care is responsible for referrals from primary care professionals. An example of this is when you see your GP who advises that you need to have an operation. Secondary care includes NHS Trusts, Mental Health Trusts, Care Trusts, Ambulance Trusts and Emergency and Urgent Care. The 1,600 NHS hospitals are overseen by 175 Acute NHS Trusts and 60 Mental Health Trusts. There are also 115 Foundation Trusts in England.

NHS Direct

NHS Direct is the national health advice line. It is available 24 hours a day, seven days a week, and 365 days a year. The service offers the opportunity for users to phone them with any health concerns, which can then be assessed over the phone and further advice given.

The service also has a comprehensive website which has an enormous amount of information and advice available for users to refer to. There is a symptom checker that you can use if you don't want to speak to someone on the phone.

Acute Trusts

These are responsible for managing hospitals and employ a large proportion of the NHS workforce. They offer specialised care in the form of regional and national centres, as well as training facilities and services in the community.

Foundation Trusts

This is a new type of NHS hospital which is tailored to the needs of the local population. They have a greater degree of financial and operational freedom than other types of NHS trust. They were introduced in April 2004.

Ambulance Trusts

These are ambulance services in England which offer an emergency ambulance system and rapid response vehicles as well as general transportation for certain types of patient to and from hospital.

Care Trusts

These trusts work within both health and social care. They operate in areas where local authorities and the NHS have agreed to work together more closely.

Primary Care Trusts

You will be seen by a service which forms part of the Primary Care Trust when you first need to consult someone about a health issue. This could be a call to NHS Direct or a visit to your dentist. The PCT controls all of the healthcare services for your local community.

Mental Health Trusts

These are Mental Health Care trusts that provide services for those with mental health problems. These can include counselling, therapy and specialist care for people suffering from severe conditions such as schizophrenia, depression and so on.

Private healthcare

Whilst we are very lucky in the UK to have a National Health Service, it is not the only option available to us.

If you are in a position to afford it, private medical care can be an excellent investment. Most people gain access to private healthcare facilities by taking out Private Medical Insurance (PMI). This type of insurance should not be confused with health cash plans, critical illness or income protection insurance.

According to the Association of British Insurers, the definition of Private Medical Insurance is 'insurance...designed to cover the costs of private medical treatment for what are commonly known as 'acute conditions' that start after your policy begins'.

For most people, the appeal of PMI is that, should they become ill, they will have access to the top consultant specialists and best treatment quickly; they will have a choice of where to have the treatment, and that the facilities in the hospitals are much more comfortable and luxurious than those in NHS hospitals.

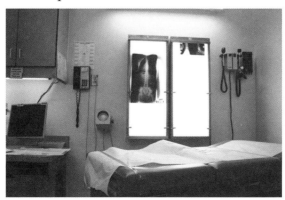

You can obtain PMI direct from the insurer, or via a broker, or from a third party such as a bank or supermarket. It can be arranged in person, over the phone, via post or on the Internet. If you are arranging your PMI via a third party, then do check whether they are independent or affiliated to one particular company as this will affect the range of products that they can offer you. Many people have PMI included as a benefit with their employment.

Policies vary widely so it is important to consider how much you are willing to spend and what you would like to be included in your cover. Some policies don't include diagnostic tests, or offer a choice of hospitals.

At the time of taking out the policy you will be asked some quite detailed questions. These are important because they form the basis for the cover you are being offered and, as previously mentioned, any pre-existing conditions are likely not to be covered.

No matter which type of policy you have, the treatment and referral process is likely to be similar. It is usual for you to see your GP in the first instance and they will then make the appropriate diagnosis. They will then make a referral to a specialist for a consultation and maybe diagnostic tests. It is usually at this point that you would contact the insurance company to make a claim.

You will then attend hospital on either an outpatient or inpatient basis. It will either be a private hospital, or private facilities within an NHS hospital. You will undergo any treatment and you will be told if you need to come back in the future.

After your treatment is finished you might be asked to attend a follow-up appointment to review your condition and the treatment you have had.

Once it has been established that you need to have some treatment, most insurance companies require you to contact them first so that they can confirm that you are covered for the treatment required. They will probably require you to keep them regularly updated so that they can continually assess your claim for validity.

Not all illnesses or conditions will be covered by the insurance, particularly any that you were already suffering from at the time of taking out the policy. PMI also rarely covers chronic conditions requiring long-term treatment such as diabetes. This sort of condition is what the NHS is designed for. PMI is for acute conditions that can be treated quickly. The types of conditions not usually covered by PMI are:

Injuries requiring treatment by Accident and Emergency.
Drug abuse related problems.
HIV/AIDS.
Pregnancy.
Sex changes.
Mobility.
Organ transplants.
Injuries sustained from participating in hazardous pursuits.
Dental treatment.
Medication and dressings.
Injuries caused by self-harming.
Infertility.
Cosmetic surgery.
Experimental treatments.
Kidney dialysis.
Injuries sustained during war.

(Source: Association of British Insurers, 2009)

Whilst private hospitals are usually extremely well equipped, they are very much intended to run alongside the NHS facilities, so will not have an Accident and Emergency department for example.

Self-pay
Whilst the vast majority of people (over seven million in the UK) choose to access private medical care via a Private Medical Insurance policy, there is an alternative. You can choose to pay for one-off treatments or procedures directly to the hospital – this is called self-pay.

Self-pay can represent a viable way to access private medical care without being tied to monthly premiums or restricted to what is covered by the policy. It is an excellent choice if you want to bypass NHS waiting lists which, even though they are not as long as they once were, are still significant enough to make people think seriously about going private.

There are several factors that you should consider when deciding whether to opt for PMI or self-pay:

Age
Medical insurance policy premiums increase the older you are. This is because older people are more likely to require medical treatment. Self-pay charges are based on the procedure required, not on your age.

Medical history
PMI does not generally cover pre-existing conditions, just illnesses that you get after your policy has started. If you want to have an operation for a condition you have suffered from for a long time then you might be better off choosing self-pay as it will most likely not be covered by PMI.

Policy exemptions
PMI will have various conditions and procedures that are not covered by the policy such as childbirth, cosmetic surgery and dental services. If you require a procedure that is not covered by PMI then it will be best to choose self-pay.

How to arrange self-pay treatment
In the first instance you will need to see your GP to arrange a referral and once you have this in place you can start to contact hospitals to get quotes for your treatment. Once a price is agreed then a contract will be drawn up which will show what is included in the price. Normally it will incorporate:

> Medical care.
> Private room.
> Operation fees.
> Drugs and dressings.
> Longer stay due to complications.

Some things will not be included – you will have to pay extra for these:

Consultation fee.
Diagnostic tests.
Anaesthetist fees.
Medication to take home.
Personal sundries such as phone calls.

Fees are usually payable before treatment goes ahead.

Our health always seems much more valuable after we lose it.

Unknown Author

Ten:
Incidents

The purpose of this section is not to scare or sound like a doom-monger. It is to raise awareness of some of the avoidable tragedies that have taken place. Each year thousands of patients die as a result of human error and we need to ask whether enough is being done to protect us. Until that time arrives there is a need to be more aware and better informed, so that we are equipped to prevent the same things happening to us or our family.

According to the independent charity Action Against Medical Accidents, a medical accident can be defined as 'where avoidable harm has been caused as a result of treatment or failure to treat appropriately'.

Medical errors happen either because we do the wrong thing (make the wrong diagnosis or give the wrong drug) or we do the right thing wrong. Often we blame 'the system' for causing errors e.g. the lack of manpower that leaves exhausted and inexperienced staff without supervision, but errors can happen in ideal circumstances and deaths can occur during routine operations, due to human error. Even for the most senior medical and nursing staff when put in very stressful situations, things can go horribly wrong.

There have been many cases recorded of medical accidents and these are just some of the stories of the victims who suffered as a result of poor treatment. By reading these stories, hopefully it will make you more aware of what can go wrong and what you need to be aware of when you or a loved one is undergoing treatment.

Robbie Powell

Robbie Powell, who was 10 years old, died in 1990 following allegations of neglectful treatment. There had been apparent delays in the treatment of his Addison's disease. There seemed to have been some inconsistencies in his medical records which Robbie's father, Will, noticed. These were reported to the police in 1994.

No less than three police investigations took place, the last one being by an external police force because the first two which had been carried out by Dyfed Powys Police were found to be institutionally incompetent.

Allegations of forgery were made against several doctors and the GMC were informed about this in 1994, which they acknowledged in 1995.

A report to the Crown Prosecution Service in 2003 concluded that there was enough evidence to prosecute these doctors for forgery and for perverting the course of justice; however, the case was not brought due to procedural problems.

The GMC indicated at the time that they would proceed with their own investigation. They reiterated this to Powys Local Health Board who formally referred the matter to the GMC themselves in December 2004.

By May 2008, an investigation by the GMC still hadn't gone ahead and they decided that because the events leading to the death of Robbie had taken place more than five years previous to them being made aware of the allegations, they would no longer be going ahead with an investigation.

Action Against Medical Accidents is currently pursuing a judicial review of the case.

A settlement was made in respect of a clinical negligence claim in 1996.

Denise Hendry

The wife of footballer Colin Hendry sadly died in 2009 after enduring several years of complications resulting from a botched liposuction procedure in 2002.

She opted to have the cosmetic procedure at Broughton Park Hospital in Preston, Lancashire, after having her fourth child. The operation went very wrong, with Mrs Hendry suffering nine punctures to her bowel and colon. This caused the onset of septicaemia and multiple organ failure and she suffered a cardiac arrest - her heart stopped for four minutes. The surgeon who operated on her voluntarily removed himself from the GMC Register but is thought to be working at a clinic in Sweden.

Mrs Hendry had to undergo corrective surgery including a 16-hour operation in May 2009. It was after this procedure that she contracted meningitis from which she did not recover.

In May 2009 she went into a coma and eventually had to be taken off of life support after having spent 12 weeks in intensive care. She died aged 43.

Arun Rees

Arun Rees was the son of Krishna Govekar and Johanne Rees. He was left brain damaged after staff waited for 90 minutes to deliver him despite his being in distress. Doctors and midwives did not spot that he was in distress and one doctor even suggested that Johanne was not in labour at all and simply needed to go to the toilet.

After his birth in November 2005 it became apparent that his brain had been starved of oxygen. Ten days later the decision was taken to turn off his life support machine.

Johanne Rees had been in the care of the Fetal Medicine Unit because her waters had broken at 18 weeks, so her pregnancy was considered high risk. At her last antenatal appointment she had been told that Arun was in the breech position and that she would need to have a caesarean section.

She was admitted to hospital at 32 weeks gestation with severe abdominal pains, but was not monitored properly, midwives missing the signs from the CTG heart readings that the baby was distressed.

After the first doctor dismissed her fears, a further 90 minutes passed before another doctor took the decision that an emergency caesarean was necessary. He was taken to the Special Care Baby Unit immediately where he was placed on a life support machine.

Arun's parents received £160,000 in compensation from the Cardiff and Vale University Health Board, which is responsible for the University Hospital of Wales where Arun was born. The hospital apologised unreservedly although they refused to admit anything had gone wrong with the management of her labour.

(Source: *The Daily Telegraph*, 2009)

Hazel Fenton

Hazel Fenton is a grandmother in her 80s, who, if it wasn't for the persistence of her daughter, would have died under a controversial NHS care plan.

Hazel had been placed onto the Liverpool Care Pathway plan (LCP) at Conquest Hospital in Hastings. The LCP is a scheme for caring for cancer patients nearing the end of their lives. She had been identified by doctors as being terminally ill and would only survive for another few days.

The LCP means that medical staff can stop administering fluids and medication to patients who are dying. The patients are then continuously sedated until the time of death.

Hazel Fenton had been admitted to hospital suffering from pneumonia and a junior doctor told Mrs Fenton's daughter, Christine Ball, that she would be placed on the LCP 'to make her more comfortable' during her final days.

Miss Ball repeatedly asked hospital staff to take her mother off the LCP and insert an artificial feeding tube. She was even approached by a nurse at one stage to be asked what she wanted to be done with her mother's body when she died.

On the day of Mrs Fenton's 80th birthday, she told her daughter that she 'didn't want to die'. Miss Ball then had to spend another 4 days persuading doctors to resume artificial feeding.

The decision to place Mrs Fenton on the LCP was taken under the Mental Capacity Act which classes food and hydration as treatment and therefore withdrawable under certain circumstances.

The LCP has been highly criticised by many including some doctors, who have seen it being used too widely in the NHS. It is possible that it has resulted in treatment being denied to patients who are not actually dying. Palliative care consultant, Peter Hargreaves, has expressed concern that patients who could make a recovery are being left to die under the plan.

At the time of writing, Hazel Fenton was being cared for in a nursing home.

(Source: *The Sunday Times*, 2009)

Dr Richard Neale

Dr Richard Neale was found guilty by the General Medical Council of 34 counts of failing to provide appropriate care and lying about his qualifications.

He started his career in London, qualifying as a doctor and becoming a member of The Royal College of Surgeons in 1970. In 1977 he emigrated to Canada where he started work at the Prince George Hospital in British Columbia.

Colleagues became alarmed at the number of complications which arose during his operations, and the blood bank were concerned at the amount of blood that was being used by him. In 1978, a 56-year-old patient, Joyce Kitchen, died after being operated on by him against the advice of the head of surgery.

After this incident he was banned in British Columbia, but moved to Toronto and started work at the Oshawa Hospital. In 1981, pregnant Geraldine Krawchuk died at the hospital after Neale gave her an overdose of the drug prostaglandin, which is used to induce labour. The drug was banned for use by the hospital, so Neale must have obtained it elsewhere. Mrs Krawchuk was given ten times the recommended dose of the drug which caused her to bleed to death. Her baby survived.

Neale was then struck off by the Ontario College of Physicians and Surgeons in 1985.

Richard Neale returned to the UK, where he started work as a consultant obstetrician and gynaecologist at the Friarage Hospital in Yorkshire, despite the GMC having been informed that he had been struck off in Canada.

He became the director of the Maternity Unit at the hospital in 1990, but left the post in 1995 due to 'concerns about his commitment' with a £100,000 severance payment and clean reference.

The reference enabled him to start work as a locum, taking up posts in Leicester and the Isle of Wight, the London Fertility Clinic, and the Portland Hospital in London.

It was suggested that Leicester Royal Infirmary contacted the GMC with concerns about Richard Neale in 1995, but that the GMC failed to respond. In 1998 the GMC announced that they were looking into two complaints against him, after which more than 60 women came forward to also complain against him. He was eventually struck off the General Medical Register in July 2000.

(Source: Department of Health, 2004)

Martin Ryan

Martin Ryan had Down's Syndrome and suffered from epilepsy. He died at the age of 43 after suffering a stroke in November 2005. He had been living in a residential home in Kingston, south west London, when the stroke happened and he was admitted to Kingston Hospital.

As a result of the stroke, he had been left unable to swallow, and was also unable to speak. Incredibly, medical staff did not take these factors into account when thinking about his nutritional needs, and no action was taken to feed him.

He spent 18 days in a hospital bed, literally starving before it was realised by medical staff that he should have had a feeding tube fitted. He was, by this time, too unwell to undergo the procedure, and sadly died eight days later having gone without food for 26 days.

The internal investigation carried out by the hospital found that doctors were under the impression that Mr Ryan was being fed by nurses through a naso-gastric tube.

The family of Martin Ryan made a complaint to the hospital and reported the case to the Healthcare Commission. The Health Ombudsman was asked to investigate Martin's death and the investigation concluded that all of the complaints made about his care should be upheld. These were:

That there were failings in stroke care.
That there were failings in clinical leadership.

That there were failings in communication and multidisciplinary team working.

That there had been a failure to feed Mr Ryan which resulted in malnutrition and starvation.

That there was an un-remedied injustice caused by maladministration in the way the trust handled Mrs Ryan's complaint.

Mr Ryan's parents were awarded £40,000 compensation.

(Sources: Mencap, 2009 and Carvel, 2009)

Emma Kemp

Emma Kemp was 26 years old and suffered from severe learning difficulties. She lived in a residential care home, but regularly spent time with her mother and grandparents.

Emma became unwell in April 2004 and over the course of about a month saw several GPs and community health workers. In May 2004 she was admitted to hospital as an emergency case, whereupon examination, a hospital doctor discovered a lump in her groin.

Tests undertaken by the hospital revealed that Emma was suffering from non-Hodgkin's lymphoma, which is a malignant tumour of the lymph system.

Consultants took the decision that there was a less than 10% chance of successfully treating the tumour and Emma was transferred to a specialist palliative care facility where she died in 2004.

Emma's mother made a complaint about her daughter's care because she felt that, firstly, her daughter's condition should have been spotted earlier than it was and that, secondly, her daughter was treated less favourably because of her learning difficulties. Mrs Kemp also felt that her initial complaint had not been handled appropriately.

The investigation into Emma's death by the Health Ombudsman did not find that the NHS had failed in its duty to her, but Emma's mother still feels that more could have been done to save her daughter.

Emma's story was included in a Mencap report entitled 'Death by Indifference' which suggested that people with learning disabilities were not getting the best treatment from the NHS. The report has led to an ongoing campaign to ensure that people with learning disabilities get equal healthcare to the rest of the population.

(Source: Parliamentary and Health Service Ombudsman, 2009)

Mark Cannon

Thirty-year-old Mark Cannon suffered from a learning disability and epilepsy. Whilst in respite care during the summer of 2003 he broke his leg and had to be admitted to Oldchurch Hospital in Romford.

It was necessary for him to have an operation on his leg, after which he collapsed, having lost 40% of his blood because the staff had forgotten to give him a blood transfusion.

The medication which controlled his epilepsy was not managed correctly, which caused him to suffer unnecessary fits.

He was not given any pain relief for his leg and was discharged in a lot of pain.

Mark was re-admitted to hospital shortly after that with renal failure. He then contracted a chest infection, had a heart attack and died of multi- organ failure.

Mark's family complained about failures in his care which prompted an investigation by the Health Ombudsman. They found that there had been shortcomings which did contribute to his early death.

(Source: Bennett, 2009)

Bethany Bowen

Five-year-old Bethany Bowen died on the operating table after a trainee surgeon tried out a new piece of equipment on her. The operation took place at the John Radcliffe Hospital in Oxford in July 2006. The device, called a morcellator, is though to have cut through her aorta.

Bethany's parents had not been told that surgeons were planning to use the morcellator during the operation. It is a fairly routine procedure and had been carried out on other members of Bethany's family previously. Bethany suffered from a hereditary condition called spherocytosis, which causes the body to produce the wrong shaped red blood cells. These are then attacked and destroyed by the spleen leading to anaemia. The only way to cure this is to remove the spleen completely.

The pathologist who carried out the post mortem on Bethany's body told the inquest that he had never seen internal injuries like these before. The results of the inquest were not conclusive, although the hospital later admitted negligence and paid her family £10,000 in compensation.

Penny Campbell

Penny Campbell was a 41-year-old journalist who died from multiple organ failure after contacting eight different doctors via an out of hours GP Service.

She died in March 2005 having made six phone calls and seen two doctors in person over the Easter Bank holiday weekend. She was not offered appropriate care because of problems in how the out of hours service was run.

On each occasion that Penny Campbell contacted doctors her case was treated as an individual episode and not looked at as a whole. She was told to call back if she didn't recover which clearly she did on several occasions. There was no system in place to ensure that doctors could easily access patient notes, which was a contributing factor to Miss Campbell's death.

During her various consultations she was diagnosed with colic, flu and a viral infection, as the doctors she spoke to failed to recognise the seriousness of her condition.

Penny Campbell had been given an injection for haemorrhoids a few days earlier, which, because she was a carrier of Group A Streptococcus, led to the bacteria being introduced into her bloodstream. Normally this infection could be adequately treated by antibiotics, provided that they are administered in time. In Penny Campbell's case they were not, which is what led to her death.

The day after the injection she had begun to feel unwell and her symptoms became progressively worse. She was suffering from a fever, a rash, and increasing abdominal pain. Her temperature was 41 degrees and she reported to doctors that she was almost unable to walk.

It was only after speaking to the eighth doctor that she was finally admitted to hospital where the urgency of her condition was realised too late to save her. She died a few hours later.

The report into the events surrounding her death found that there had been a 'major systems failure'. Her partner is pursuing legal action over her death.

Jimmy Stewart

Jimmy Stewart was left badly brain damaged, and in need of 24 hour care after attempts to resuscitate him at Northern Ireland's biggest hospital went badly wrong.

Mr Stewart was originally admitted to hospital with a chest infection but he developed pneumonia and was admitted to Intensive Care. After 12 days he was moved to a general ward where he was placed in a side room because he was considered an infection risk, having contracted superbugs four times whilst in hospital.

Mr Stewart suffered a cardiac arrest after his oxygen supply became disconnected. An alarm, which should have notified staff, was not audible from the nurses' station, so there was a delay in reaching him. When staff did reach him they were unaware that he was a tracheotomy patient and had to breathe through a tube in his throat. They began resuscitating him via his mouth and nose, which meant that air was going into his stomach instead of his lungs.

Mr Stewart's brain was being deprived of oxygen for the entire episode which resulted in the brain damage.

An investigation into the incident found that there had been an inadequate level of care and monitoring of Mr Stewart prior to his cardiac arrest. There was also a failure to react to the deterioration in his condition. Staff did not notice that his oxygen supply tube had become disconnected and that there was an unnecessary delay in resuscitating him.

Other findings were that the alarm was practically inaudible outside of his room and his tracheotomy tube had not been downsized as per recommendations. Several doses of a drug that he had been prescribed had not been administered, and observations were not carried out as frequently as they should have been.

The Belfast Trust in charge of the hospital has accepted that there were failings in Mr Stewart's care.

Lee Nicholls

Teenager Lee Nicholls died after suffering a brain haemorrhage which had been caused by an aneurysm. He was admitted to hospital suffering from double vision, headaches and vomiting.

Doctors did not take the aneurysm into account and said that he was suffering from meningitis for which he was given antibiotics. Lee was given a lumbar puncture which should have been tested for a substance which would have indicated bleeding on the brain but this did not happen.

Lee was discharged from hospital, but after a few weeks he collapsed and had to be put on to a life support machine. He died after suffering another haemorrhage, which had been missed by doctors, despite having undergone two separate CT scans.

At the inquest into his death, the coroner criticised four areas of his treatment – the misdiagnosis as meningitis, the failure to transfer him to a specialist neurosurgery unit, the failure to test the spinal fluid and the failure to ensure that a neurologist examined the images from the CT scan.

Jo Dowling

Jo Dowling, 25 years old, was admitted to Milton Keynes Hospital with a letter from her GP stating that she had meningitis. However doctors and nurses said that Jo had only a mild infection. Jo sent text messages to her mother and friend saying that she was getting worse. She died 14 hours after being admitted.

An inquest heard that a simple course of antibiotics would have saved her life. The inquest heard there were only two doctors on duty to cover the entire hospital overnight.

Rosemary McFarlane

Gross failure and neglect contributed to the death of a grandmother of five, a coroner ruled. Rosemary McFarlane, 64, a patient in Heartlands Hospital in Birmingham, died after 'gross failures' by NHS doctors who injected her lungs with a chemical that was ten times the recommended strength, a coroner ruled. Mrs McFarlane spent ten days in 'burning agony' after receiving the lethal dose, during what should have been a routine procedure.

Carla McAdam

Carla McAdam, 28 years old, was treated five times at the Ulster Hospital, Dundonald, and died after doctors failed to diagnose an 'ectopic pregnancy'. The coroner criticised the absence of dialogue between consultants and nurses at the hospital and concluded that at no point did the doctors step back and ask, 'Why is Carla ill'?

Mistakes are a way of life for doctors

Apart from the very serious cases that hit the headlines because they involve children or celebrities, or particularly vulnerable people according to many within the medical profession, there are constant mistakes made by doctors which colleagues may well be aware of but, because of the very closed nature of the medical profession, they don't tend to report them unless they absolutely have to.

A substantial percentage of the population has a fear of flying, yet the odds of dying in hospital as a result of human error are 33,000 times greater than the risk of dying in an air crash. This was stated by the late Dr. Tom Chalmers, medical researcher, who also said, 'If doctors died with their patients, they'd take a great deal more care'.

The book *The Incompetent Doctor* by Marilynn M. Rosenthal examines exactly how the medical profession regulates itself and describes some shocking incidents involving doctors.

> A series of complaints against an orthopaedic surgeon who failed to diagnose a broken back and left the patient sitting up in a wheelchair.
> Doctors being able to carry on practising for years whilst addicted to drugs or alcohol with the knowledge of their peers.
> Doctors carrying out procedures that fell outside of their remit.
> Doctors failing to diagnose serious conditions such as meningitis.
> Doctors mis-prescribing medication.

Surgeons carrying out operations on the wrong part of the body.
Patients being given the wrong blood group.
Doctors who are impaired by some sort of ill health which affects them physically or mentally.

The book notes that doctors are not trained to ask for help because it is like admitting that they are incompetent, therefore those doctors who actually are incompetent have a tendency to isolate themselves until they make such a major mistake that it forces them out into the open.

(Source: Rosenthal, 1995)

In a Government Report, Sube Banertee, Professor of Mental Health and Ageing at the Institute of Psychiatry at King's College London, stated that up to 1,800 elderly dementia patients are dying each year from wrongly prescribed anti-psychotic drugs. He said that often these powerful drugs are being used unnecessarily.

Only around 36,000 of the 180,000 people currently on the drugs in the UK are getting any benefit from them, leaving 144,000 people taking these drugs with dangerous and life-threatening side effects. In most cases these 144,000 elderly people are wrongly prescribed the drugs as a chemical restraint.

Anti-psychotic medicines are officially licensed to treat people with schizophrenia, but are available as an option to treat more serious symptoms seen in dementia patients in care homes and hospitals. However the scandalous over-prescribing of anti-psychotic drugs for dementia patients leads to an estimated 1,800 deaths a year.

A three year study published in the Lancet Neurology found people taking the drugs for long periods were twice as likely to die early as those not taking them. Other studies have shown that people taking these drugs were three times more likely to have a stroke.

Side effects include dizziness and unsteadiness, which can lead to falls and injuries. Other side effects are shaking, restlessness, social withdrawal and severe sensitivity reactions. Dementia patients on these drugs can have terrific nightmares, stop eating and become bedridden. What a horrific way for an elderly person in a care home to end their life.

If a dementia patient, with behaviour problems, in a care home is on anti-psychotic medication, this 'chemical cosh' makes the dementia sufferer easier to manage and makes life much easier for the care staff of the care home.

Many people who suffer from mental illness are also being chemically restrained because it makes life a lot easier for those responsible for their welfare.

Treating the most vulnerable members of society in this despicable way is much less expensive in the short term than providing adequate numbers of properly trained carers. We don't treat or regard people with dementia or people with mental disabilities with anywhere near the kind of respect that they deserve.

It is terrible that people with dementia and mental illness are being 'chemically coshed' and left to live in a trance-like state for the rest of their lives. Staff in care homes and hospitals should challenge the doctors who are prescribing these anti-psychotic drugs. They should be vigilant that the people in their care are not being given medication they don't require and they should see to it that each individual in their care, and that individual's medication, is regularly reviewed.

If you have a relative who has dementia or a mental disability, living at home, in a care home, or in a hospital, educate yourself regarding the medication they are receiving, question their doctor as to the need for the medication, see that their medication is regularly reviewed and be present at the review.

Jeremy Wright, chairman of the all party Parliamentary Group on Dementia, told BBC Radio 4's Today programme: 'We need to involve family members and friends and loved ones much more in the decision to prescribe and the decision to keep prescribing these drugs'.

The medical profession tend to use drugs first, because it takes less time than other means of diagnosis or treatment. Prescribing drugs is handy and quick for doctors.

Thousands of people are dying each year as a result of being prescribed the wrong medication. People are dying while pharmaceutical companies make piles of money. Indeed anti-psychotic drugs are big earners for the drug companies. Pharmacology is primarily a money-making business and the drug companies will always find ways to encourage doctors to continue prescribing their drugs.

It is health that is real wealth and not pieces of gold and silver.

Mahatma Gandhi

Eleven: Being Assertive

Assertiveness can be defined as the ability to speak up for ourselves and to say what we are feeling when the need arises. It is a way of giving our own needs and rights the same importance as the needs of other people which is essential for our own well-being, particularly in a healthcare situation.

Often people feel unable to act in an assertive manner because they fear the consequences of their assertive behaviour. In a doctor-patient situation, many of us might feel that if we speak up the doctor might talk down to us or make us feel small or stupid.

In reality, however, assertive behaviour is normally treated with respect, so you will probably be pleasantly surprised with how the doctor responds to you. They will be able to see that you respect and care for yourself because you are willing to stand up for yourself and tell them what your thoughts are.

Being assertive is not about being aggressive. It is the middle ground between passivity and aggression. If you behave too passively then you are at risk of only getting what other people want for you or themselves and this, of course, includes medical treatment.

Don't worry if you are not sure how to be assertive, because there are lots of hints and tips available to help you. It is a skill that can be learned and it doesn't mean completely changing your personality.

Being assertive means staying in control of your emotions. Because of the way we have been taught by society to behave towards doctors, sometimes we can feel intimidated by them. This can prevent us from communicating with them in the right way to ensure that we understand our treatment.

If you are not used to behaving in an assertive manner it can feel like a difficult thing to do at first, but the more you assert yourself, the easier it will become. Assertiveness is a really great communication tool to have in all areas of your life. Assertiveness can help boost self-esteem which can be a factor in illnesses such as depression, so is a really useful skill to learn.

If you don't feel comfortable with what the doctor has told you, then you have every right to a second opinion (or even a third) and you should not be afraid to ask for one. There is nothing to stop you seeking a specialist yourself; the information is readily available on the Internet.

You should expect and demand quality in the care and treatment you receive. Don't be concerned about staying quiet and being polite – this is your health.

Become as informed as you possibly can about your condition. Knowledge is power. You should take the time to thoroughly research your illness and any treatments that are being suggested to you and try to compare different options to see if there are any differences.

Find out independently about drugs and their side effects. You can also look up hospital league tables to compare waiting times, infection rates and other important data. You can also compare data on doctors, specialists and consultants.

Keep up to date with the medical press around the world. You never know when there might be a new treatment available that your doctor might not have become aware of. Remember they have to generalise a lot of the time and might not always have your particular case in mind. Take responsibility for bringing the information to their attention.

Take responsibility for your own health. The doctor is not the be all and end all.

Take the lead. There is nothing wrong with asking questions – as many as you need to ask until you understand fully what the doctor is talking about. Don't let the doctor rush you.

You are the only one who truly cares about you, so double check what your doctor is telling you. They are not always right and don't always have your best interests in mind. Be involved in your treatment. Don't just lie back and let the medical profession do things to you. Keep a record of your symptoms, treatment, appointments and drugs.

Involve your family and close friends. Get their opinions on your condition and treatment. If you are in hospital ask them to bring you fresh fruit and drinks to supplement what is available to you in hospital.

If you are in hospital and are concerned about the level of care you are receiving - for example you don't feel that you are getting the food that you need – speak to the nursing staff. Don't assume that they will know about any special dietary needs or whether you need assistance with eating.

You can check with your local council for details on hospital food hygiene inspections. If they don't want to give you the information straight away then you can use a Freedom of Information request.

Ways to improve your assertiveness

Body language
Assertive behaviour is closely linked to the way that we hold and move our bodies. A typical example of passive body language would be to hunch your shoulders and avoid eye contact, whereas clenching of the fists and a glaring expression would portray aggressiveness. On the other hand, the assertive individual would be standing upright, but in a relaxed manner, keeping their hands open and looking people in the eye.

By looking at our own body language in the mirror, and by consciously trying to adopt the different passive, aggressive and assertive stances, we can become more aware of how we are projecting ourselves to others and make sure that we are giving across the impression that we want to.

Communication
The way that we communicate can also have a big impact on whether we are perceived as being assertive or not. To communicate effectively it is important to ensure that you can demonstrate knowledge of the situation at hand (i.e. your condition or medication), that you can also

communicate the way that you feel about it, and that you can clearly explain what you want and need from the situation.

In a doctor-patient situation it will be helpful for you to be prepared prior to the appointment. Think honestly about what your own feelings are about the situation so that you can communicate them succinctly.

Whilst talking to the doctor stay calm and stick to the point and use some written notes if necessary. If the doctor says something that you are not sure about or don't understand then don't be afraid to ask for clarification. If you feel that the doctor is not getting the point of what you are saying, then stay calm and reiterate what you want to say.

(Source: BUPA, 2008)

Assertiveness techniques

There are three key assertiveness techniques that can be really helpful to learn. You can then use them as a tool to communicate more effectively not just with your doctor but with everyone that you have to deal with in life.

Broken Record

The Broken Record techniques get their name from the days when vinyl records were our main medium for listening to music. Occasionally, the stylus of the record player would get stuck and the same bit of the record would play over and over again.

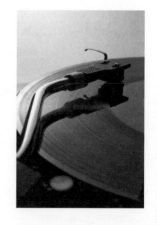

As an assertiveness technique, Broken Record involves repeating a request repeatedly until a resolution or compromise is reached. A good example of using this during a medical consultation might be if you found that the doctor was skirting around your requests for a second opinion. If you keep on reiterating your desire for a second opinion then the doctor is going to find it increasingly difficult to change the subject or ignore your wishes.

Fogging

Fogging refers to an assertiveness technique which many people use to block out negativity.

If you are facing criticism from another person, this technique is based on agreeing that the probability of what they are saying is correct. By allowing them to continue criticising you without a reaction on your part it deflates them somewhat and expends their energy more quickly.

Suggestions of responses that you can use to the other person who is criticising you include:

> "Yes I think that too…"
> "I agree with you…"
> "I do do that sometimes, don't I…"?

With this technique you are actually acknowledging that there might be some truth in the criticism, but because you are vocalising it yourself, there is less impact.

Negative assertion

This is a technique for dealing with criticism without letting it get to you. By simply agreeing with all or part of what the critic (the doctor in this case) might be saying to you (you haven't been sticking to your diet or you haven't taken your medication correctly) it then stops the criticism from feeling like a personal attack and turns it to something that you admit and are in control of.

DESC scripting

DESC stands for:

> Describe.
> Express.
> Specify.
> Consequences.

It is a way of putting across complaints or requests and is very effective.

You Describe the issue, Express your feelings about it, Specify what you would like to see done about it, and the Consequences are what will happen as a result which can be either negative or positive.

(Source: Ormondroyd, 2004)

The book *When I Say No I Feel Guilty* by Manuel Smith, which was published in 1975, contained a 'Bill of Assertive Rights' which is useful to refer to in order to remind yourself of what you have the right to say, do and feel.

> You have the right to judge your own behaviour, thoughts, and emotions, and to take the responsibility for their initiation and consequences upon yourself.
>
> You have the right to offer no reasons or excuses for justifying your behaviour.
>
> You have the right to judge if you are responsible for finding solutions to other people's problems.
>
> You have the right to change your mind.
>
> You have the right to make mistakes and be responsible for them.
>
> You have the right to say, "I don't know".
>
> You have the right to be independent of the goodwill of others before coping with them.
>
> You have the right to be illogical in making decisions.
>
> You have the right to say, "I don't understand".
>
> You have the right to say, "I don't care".

(Source: Smith, 1975)

Legislation

Make sure you are aware of any legislation which might affect you as a patient. At the time of writing, the following laws can all relate to you as a patient on the NHS, whether it is with regard to your care or the confidentiality of your information.

Mental Capacity Act 2005

This legislation is relevant because it deals with our ability or inability to make decisions and makes specific reference to provision of medical treatment by the NHS, with particular provisions for emergency situations where treatment is required.

Data Protection Act 1998

Your medical records are protected by the provisions of the Data Protection Act. Anyone who handles them has to abide by certain principles set out in the act and there are serious penalties for non-compliance.

This act also gives you the right to access your medical records. You can do this by writing to the organisation holding the records and making an official request. There is usually a charge.

Human Rights Act 1998

Based on the European Convention on Human Rights, this act sets out a number of rights and freedoms that all citizens of the United Kingdom are entitled to. Some of them that might be relevant in the course of dealing with medical services are:

The right to life.
The right to respect for private and family life.
The right to freedom of thought, conscience and religion and freedom to express your beliefs.
The right not to be discriminated against in respect of these rights and freedoms.

If your rights are breached then you can pursue legal action.

Freedom of Information Act 2000

Public authorities, including the NHS, hold a great deal of information that it may be of interest to access. The Freedom of Information Act provides the mechanisms for us to do so. Public bodies have certain obligations under the act and when a request is received they have to follow a set procedure.

Authorities that fail to meet their obligations under the act can be subjected to enforcement action.

Fond of doctors, little health.

Fond of lawyers, little wealth.

Proverb

Twelve: Healthy Mindset and Lifestyle

At the end of the day, prevention is better than cure. We need to understand our bodies and our health and we need to lead healthier lifestyles. Don't treat your health as a lottery, gambling that you will remain in good health throughout your life. Take the steps now to live a healthier life, take care of your body and insure yourself against future health issues. Life is for enjoying, not to be endured in pain or suffering from an avoidable illness.

We should all take ultimate responsibility for, and never take chances with, our health.

Diet and exercise are important for the whole family. Educate your children about how to take care of themselves.

Nutrition

Good nutrition is very important – we should all be choosing the right balance of foods in our diet to help us to stay healthy. Some people think that healthy cooking is expensive, complicated and the dishes tasteless, but this is simply not the case.

A healthy diet should be filled with a variety of foods from all of the major food groups – fruits and vegetables, starches like bread, pasta and rice, and protein from meat, fish, eggs and pulses. No single food can provide for all of our nutritional needs, so it is essential that we include a wide range in our diet.

According to Cancer Research UK, approximately one quarter of cancer deaths have been caused by unhealthy diet and obesity.

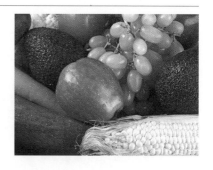

Fruit and vegetables
Fruits and vegetables are full of vitamins, minerals and fibre, and they are also low in calories. Include some form of fruit or vegetable into every meal and make them the first thing you reach for when you want a snack.

Aim to eat five portions of fruit and vegetables every day. They can be fresh, frozen, tinned, dried or juice. To give you an idea of portion sizes:

One portion is:
> 1 apple, pear, banana or orange.
> 2 plums.
> Half a grapefruit.
> 1 slice of melon.
> 3 heaped tablespoons of any vegetable.
> 3 heaped tablespoons of beans or pulses.
> 3 heaped tablespoons of fruit salad.
> 1 heaped tablespoon of dried fruit.
> 1 handful of grapes.
> Small bowl of salad.
> 150ml glass of fruit juice.

The World Health Organisation estimates that nearly 3 million deaths every year are caused by a lack of fruit and vegetables in the diet. Including plenty of fruit and vegetables in the diet can fight against illnesses such as gastrointestinal cancer, heart disease and stroke.

Green vegetables such as broccoli, spinach and cabbage are rich in minerals such as magnesium and zinc and help to strengthen the blood and respiratory systems. Sweet vegetables are a natural way of including sweetness in your diet which will help reduce cravings for cakes, biscuits and sweets.

Sweet potatoes, carrots and sweet corn are good examples. When cooking vegetables, don't overcook them and use as little water as possible. Why not try steaming your veggies?

Fruit contains natural sugars, vitamins and antioxidants. Aim to include a wide variety of fruits into your diet. Pineapples contain bromelin which breaks down artosclerotic plaques. Brightly coloured fruits and vegetables tend to contain much higher concentrations of vitamins, minerals and antioxidants. Watch out for fruit juices that contain added sugar and tinned fruit that comes in sugary syrup.

Don't store fruit and vegetables for a long time; eat them as soon as possible after purchase. If you have cut something like a cucumber then cover and chill it straight away so the nutrients are retained. Avoid keeping food hot for too long as this causes vitamin levels to drop. You can help the environment and support your local economy by purchasing your fruit and vegetables at local markets and farm shops.

Ideas for getting your five a day

Breakfast time
    Add dried fruit to your breakfast cereal.
    Have half a grapefruit.
    Drink a glass of fruit juice.

Lunch time
    Have a bowl of salad.
    Have a banana sandwich.
    Have some fruit salad.

Evening meal
    Add extra vegetables to your curry, stir fry or casserole.
    Serve two vegetables with your meat.

Carbohydrates
Carbohydrates should be wholegrain wherever possible and should make up about one third of the food you eat. Wholegrain varieties contain more fibre and nutrients.

Carbohydrates are an important source of energy and also contain fibre, iron, and calcium and B vitamins. They break down in the body to sugars which fuel our muscles and brain.

You should aim to include one portion of carbohydrate food with each meal – for example toast for breakfast, a jacket potato at lunchtime, some rice with dinner. Contrary to popular belief, carbohydrates are not really fattening. Our bodies digest carbohydrates quite slowly so they make us feel fuller for longer.

There are, however, good and bad carbs. White flour and rice and refined sugar are highly processed and have been stripped of their nutrients. They digest too rapidly and can contribute to hypoglycaemia and diabetes.

By sticking to wholegrain flour, rice, and pasta your body will digest them more slowly and you will feel fuller for longer. Wholegrains are a rich source of antioxidants and phytochemicals, which can protect against cancer, heart disease and diabetes.

To make sure you get more of the healthy starches you need in your diet you can:

> Have more rice and pasta, and less sauce.
> Have more potatoes and vegetables, and less meat.
> Add pulses to your casseroles and curries.
> Choose thick sliced bread.
> Try brown rice.
> Mix wholegrain cereal with your usual one.
> Have porridge for breakfast.

Fibre

Our bodies obtain fibre from plant foods such as fruit, vegetables and grains. Fibre is essential for maintaining a healthy digestive system.

There are two kinds of fibre – soluble and insoluble. Soluble fibre is found in oats, fruit and beans. It can dissolve in water and

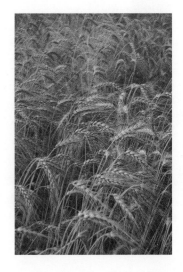

lowers blood fats, whilst maintaining blood sugar levels. Insoluble fibre passes straight through the digestive system and is found in whole grains and vegetables. It stops constipation and keeps our bowels healthy. This type of fibre also makes us feel full for longer.

We should all aim to incorporate around 20g to 30g of fibre in our diet every day.

Healthy sources of carbohydrates and fibre include:

Bread – remember to choose wholegrain.
Potatoes.
Squash.
Breakfast cereals – remember to choose wholegrain.
Beans and pulses.
Couscous.
Maize.

Protein
Our bodies need protein as it helps us to grow and repair our cells, tissues and organs. Protein is made from amino acids of which there are 20 different kinds. Some of them are known as essential amino acids.

Complete protein sources incorporate all of the 20 amino acids in one food. Meat, fish, poultry, milk and eggs fall into this category.

An incomplete protein source does not provide all 20 amino acids.

Complementary proteins are foods that combined together will provide all of the necessary amino acids. Rice and beans are a good example of this.

One of the best sources of protein is fish; it contains lots of vitamins and minerals and can be fresh, frozen, or canned. Try and incorporate a minimum of two portions of fish into your diet every week, with at least one being oily fish. These are particularly high in Omega 3 fatty acids which are good for our hearts. Oily fish would be salmon, mackerel, trout, sardines, pilchards and eels.

Alternative protein sources include nuts, beans and soya. These are excellent sources for vegetarians.

Fat

Fat is used by the body to form cell membranes; it is also oxidised for energy and can be stored by the body for later use. The fat in food is what makes us feel full and satisfied.

Avoid consuming too much in the way of saturated fats and sugar. Whilst we all need some fat in our diet, too much of the wrong sort of fat can be very bad for our health.

Nutrition Facts / Val
Per 1/2 package (85 g) / pour 1/2 e
1/2 package prepared / 1/2 emballa
Amount
Teneur
Calories / Calories
Fat / Lipides 4.5 g*   % Daily Value
Saturates / saturés 2.5 g
+ Trans / trans 0.2 g
Cholesterol / Cholestérol 15 mg
Sodium / Sodium 870 mg
Carbohydrate / Glucides 55 g
Fibre / Fibres 3 g
Sugars /

Saturated fat and trans fats are the ones we want to avoid as they increase the cholesterol levels in the blood which can increase the chances of developing heart disease. Saturated fats are generally found in foods such as sausages, pies, meat with visible fat, hard cheese, butter, lard, pastries, cakes, biscuits and cream.

Trans fats are known to be particularly harmful and are found in some margarines, sweets, biscuits and crisps. They are created by a process called hydrogenation which is when liquid vegetable oil is heated in the presence of hydrogen gas.

Consuming unsaturated fats, on the other hand, actually lowers blood cholesterol levels. There are two types of unsaturated fats – monounsaturated and polyunsaturated fats.

Monounsaturated fats are found in plant oils, nuts and seeds. Mediterranean style diets tend to be rich in these sorts of fat.

Polyunsaturated fats are rich in Omega 3 and Omega 6 fatty acids which our bodies do not produce. Sunflower and corn oils are rich in these fats.

Foods that are high in unsaturated fats include nuts and seeds, vegetable oils, oily fish and avocados.

You can check the labels on foods to work out whether something is high or low in fat. Generally speaking, more than 20g of fat per 100g could be considered high fat, whereas anything below 3g of fat per 100g is low in fat. Between these amounts is a medium level of fat.

Saturated fats will be shown separately on the label with over 5g per 100g considered high, and less than 1.5g per 100g low.

Try and keep your fat intake to no more than 30% of your total calorie consumption.

Sugar
Sugar can be found in sweets, biscuits and cakes as well as fizzy drinks. Most of us consume far too much sugar. Not only does sugar contribute to weight gain but it also causes tooth decay.

The sugar content of a food will be stated on the label. The list of ingredients always starts with what are the most prevalent ingredients, so if sugar is near to the top of the list then you can be confident that the food in question is high in sugar.

The nutritional content label will also show carbohydrates of which sugars with more than 15g per 100g is high and low is 5g or less per 100g.

Minerals

Salt
Don't have too much salt in your diet. We shouldn't consume more than about 6g per day, which sounds a lot, but many foods have a salt content which is much higher than you might think, so even if you don't add it to your food, you can still be at risk of ingesting too much salt.

The main effect of having too much salt is an increase in blood pressure which can lead to heart disease or stroke.

Check nutritional labels – a high salt content would be anything over 1.5g per 100g and a low salt content would be 0.3g per 100g.

Why not season your food using herbs instead?

Potassium
Lowers blood pressure and too little can cause heart arrhythmias.

Magnesium
Is used by the nervous system.

Calcium
Is important for bones, teeth and the nervous system. Insufficient calcium can cause osteoporosis. The best source of calcium is dairy products such as milk, cheese and yoghurt.

Iron

Is used to form red blood cells which transport oxygen around the body. Insufficient iron can result in anaemia and too much iron can be extremely dangerous.

Copper

Is an essential nutrient.

Zinc

Is for the skin and immune system.

Chromium

Is used to process carbohydrates.

Selenium

Helps the body to produce antioxidants. One and a half Brazil nuts per day will provide sufficient selenium for your body.

(Source: Paul, 2009)

Your weight

Maintaining a healthy weight is a great way of taking care of yourself. If you are overweight it can lead to heart disease and diabetes, and being underweight can also cause significant health problems.

Weight gain happens when we eat more than our bodies need, with the extra energy being stored as fat.

If you do find that you are overweight then there are plenty of weight loss resources available to help you. Alternatively you can just choose to make a few lifestyle changes such as stopping eating when you are full, choosing low fat and low sugar food options where you can, and increasing your activity levels.

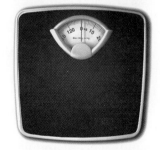

Don't ever resort to a crash diet; it is much better to lose the weight gradually at a rate of 1 to 2 lbs per week until you get to your ideal weight.

Exercise

Exercise should play a part in everyone's life, regardless of your age. All the available evidence shows that people who are physically active lessen their risks of developing serious diseases such as diabetes and heart disease, or suffering a stroke.

Exercise is also good for our mental health. Ideas of activities you can try include swimming, running, cycling, walking; even gardening and housework can help to keep you fit. Exercising can use up any excess calories and help us lose weight. It is recommended that all of us do at least 30 minutes of physical activity five days a week.

Setting yourself a challenge of a daily amount of activity is a great way to motivate yourself. A recommended way of doing this is to aim to walk 10,000 steps a day. You can track your progress by purchasing an inexpensive pedometer. Some good ways to fit more steps into your day are:

Get off the bus one stop earlier than usual.
Walk around the kitchen whilst cooking.
Walk to the train station instead of driving.
Walk to the local shops instead of driving to a superstore.
Do the school run on foot.
Go for a walk instead of having a cup of tea and a biscuit.
Take the dog for a walk.

To make walking more interesting you could find a walking partner so you have someone to talk to or get an MP3 player so you can listen to music or podcasts whilst you are walking.

Water

Drink lots of water. We need it to prevent dehydration and should be downing about two litres a day.

Our bodies are 75% water so it makes sense that we need to drink lots of it. It helps to flush waste and toxins out of our systems.

Alcohol

Whilst a little of what you fancy does you good, you should certainly keep control of your alcohol intake. Drinking too much can seriously damage your liver. Alcohol is also very high in calories and can damage the muscles of your heart.

Researchers have established that there are nine different types of drinker:

De-stress drinkers – they drink to calm down and relax.

Conformist drinkers – they visit pubs regularly and drink as a way of belonging.

Boredom drinkers – typically women, they drink alone to pass the time.

Depressed drinkers – they drink for comfort and security.

Re-bonding drinkers – they drink to connect with those close to them.

Community drinkers – they drink amongst large groups of friends.

Hedonistic drinkers – they drink to get drunk several times a week.

Macho drinkers – they drink to feel in control.

Border dependents – their pub is a home from home.

Do you recognise yourself in any of these types?

The current recommended guidelines for men and women's consumption of alcohol state that men should consume no more than three or four units of alcohol per day and women should stick to two or three. You should be aware that units of alcohol are dependent on the size of the drink and the strength of the alcohol concentration.

It is a good idea to keep an alcohol diary to assess whether you might be drinking too much. Some indications that you might have a problem with drinking are that:

You always need a drink.

You get into trouble when drinking.

People warn you that you are drinking too much.

Some of the problems that can be caused by alcohol include:

Addiction - feeling the need to drink every day.

Depression – alcohol changes brain chemistry.

Memory problems – alcohol affects your memory.

Increased cancer risk – particularly mouth, throat, breast and bowel cancers.

Heart problems – drinking can cause high blood pressure.

Liver damage - alcohol can cause serious liver problems such as cirrhosis.

Stomach problems – alcohol can cause gastritis.

Fertility problems – alcohol can cause reduced sexual performance.

If you think that you might need help with your drinking then it is a good idea to go and see your GP in the first instance. As long as you are honest with them they can assess the help you need which might include medication to help you stop drinking. They will also be able to help you find a local alcohol support group such as Alcoholics Anonymous.

Whilst it is important to be aware of the risks and not to drink too much, a small amount of alcohol can be beneficial. Research has suggested that a regular glass of red wine can help to protect against heart disease.

(Source: British Heart Foundation)

Breakfast
Considered to be the most important meal of the day, breakfast is a must for a healthy lifestyle. Eating breakfast can get your metabolism going and gives your body the rest of the day to work the calories off.

Eating habits
Don't rush your food. Chew your food slowly so you can really enjoy it. Eat in a relaxing atmosphere and not in front of the TV or on the move.

Listen to your body and only eat if you are really hungry. You might actually be dehydrated rather than hungry for food.

Try eating smaller more frequent meals to keep your metabolism going and to keep cravings away.

Health in general

Be vigilant about your health. During the course of your life you will from time to time be invited to undergo different types of health screening and testing.

Health screening is organised by the UK National Screening Committee who manage a variety of national health screening programmes. These include:

Antenatal screening during pregnancy – this checks for conditions such as Down's Syndrome.

Newborn screening – this checks for hearing impairments, cystic fibrosis, and other conditions.

Childhood screening – height, weight, vision and hearing.

Diabetic retinopathy screening – for all diabetics aged over 12.

Cervical cancer screening – for all women over 25.

Breast cancer screening – for all women over 50.

Bowel cancer screening – for all adults over 60.

Health testing is usually carried out on an ad-hoc basis by your doctor or nurse and can include cholesterol and blood pressure tests.

Don't skip checkups such as breast exams and cervical smears, they are really important.

By taking a holistic approach to your health which incorporates your mind, body and spirit, you can achieve a real sense of well-being.

Relaxation

It can be very beneficial to learn some relaxation techniques. Relaxing properly can help to release tension in your muscles, lower your blood pressure, and slow your breathing and heart rate. Relaxation techniques can be used to treat and manage a number of different conditions such as:

Anger.
Anxiety.
Cardiac problems.
Depression.

Headaches.
High Blood Pressure.
Insomnia.
Pain.
Stress.

Meditation

Meditation is a specific relaxation technique and is a natural way of promoting physical and mental well-being. It reduces stress and helps you to focus and relax. Meditation can be as simple as sitting quietly for a few minutes; alternatively there are specific meditation techniques that you can teach yourself to achieve specific states.

Yoga

This ancient discipline is a wonderful way of harmonising your mind and body. The philosophy of yoga originated around 5,000 years ago in India. It can be practised by anyone and all can benefit from it. Yoga involves exercises which stretch the body, making it more flexible the more you practise. The best way to start practising yoga is to find a class with a qualified teacher who can take you through the basic poses.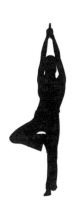

Your environment

By making your home, or at least part of it, into a peaceful, relaxing sanctuary, you will be able to slip into a relaxed state much more easily.

Candles can create a relaxing ambience and the flame of a candle can be a useful meditation tool. Choose some art that you find beautiful to put on display. Incorporate water into your surroundings – the sound of trickling water can be very relaxing, so why not invest in a small, indoor water feature, or maybe even a CD of water sounds.

Use lighting in a creative way to generate a cosy, relaxing atmosphere - pretty lamps, coloured bulbs or fairy lights can all create a lovely light effect. All of these things, together with music, comfortable furnishings and pleasant aromas will help you find relaxation whenever you wish.

Natural remedies and treatments

Try to stay away from unnecessary drugs. Even over the counter painkillers can be bad for you; research shows that many people suffer headaches from overusing painkillers. Why not try using homeopathic medicines, aromatherapy and flower remedies for minor ailments? Some of the alternative therapies available include:

Acupuncture

This ancient Chinese practice is based on the principle of Qi energy which flows along the meridians of the body. Practitioners insert fine needles at specific points in order to release blockages. It can be used in the treatment of asthma, addiction problems, arthritis, depression, anxiety, high or low blood pressure and digestive problems.

Aromatherapy

Based on the premise that pure plant oils have therapeutic properties, aromatherapy uses them to help with emotional and physical ailments. The oils can be massaged into the skin or inhaled so that the body can enjoy the healing properties.

Crystal Healing

The theory behind this treatment is that there is an interaction between the vibrational structure of the crystal and the energy within the human body and that this interaction helps to set off self-healing processes within the body.

Herbal medicine

Many modern day medicines are derived from medicinal herbs, but they have been diluted or only a part of them used. Herbal medicines are based on the whole plant and are available to treat a wide variety of conditions including depression, headaches and digestive disorders.

Homeopathy

This works on the principle that whatever causes us to be unwell can also make us better when we are ill. Homeopathic medicines are highly diluted and are available to treat many different ailments.

Hypnotherapy

By using psychotherapy and counselling methods alongside hypnosis, it is possible to induce deep relaxation and relieve certain symptoms.

Magnet Therapy

Magnets are thought to be able to relieve symptoms such as muscular aches and pains, headaches and insomnia. The treatment is controversial and not suitable for people fitted with a pacemaker or who are having radiotherapy treatment.

Massage Therapy

Massage involves the manipulation of soft tissue for therapeutic means. Aches and pains and stress are ideal for treatment by massage therapy.

Osteopathy

An osteopath will manipulate the spine and muscles as a way of improving balance and mobility. This type of therapy is widely respected and can be available on the NHS in certain areas.

Reiki

This Japanese technique involves the placing of hands on certain areas of the body. Through this it is thought that spiritual energy is channelled, thereby healing the spirit and physical body.

Reflexology

This is a deep massage of the hands or feet which relaxes the whole body and breaks up crystal deposits which form at the nerve endings.

Shiatsu

Shiatsu is based on the same principles as acupuncture but involves pressure rather than needles to release energy blockages.

Mind/body connection

It is well recognised these days that there is a strong link between how we feel emotionally and our physical well-being. Some of the best work in this field comes from the following authors.

Louise Hay

Louise Hay wrote the books *Heal Your Body* and *You Can Heal your Life* and was one of the first practitioners to recognise this and teach a philosophy of using affirmations and visualisations to maintain good health. She was able to put her own teachings into practice when she herself was diagnosed with cancer and is still alive to tell the tale today. She started up her own publishing company called Hay House which publishes self-help books.

Deepak Chopra

Deepak Chopra is a qualified medical doctor but has become famous for his work on mind/body medicine. He has published a wealth of books on the subject including *Perfect Health and Return to Wholeness* which is an holistic guide to cancer.

Don't smoke

Even if you take all of the steps previously mentioned you will really be wasting your time health-wise if you smoke. Smoking can cause many illnesses including lung and other cancers with around 114,000 people dying every year from smoking-related illness.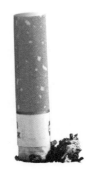

The tobacco in cigarettes releases up to 400 different toxins as it burns. The most dangerous ones are:

> Tar – this is known to cause cancer.
> Nicotine – this addictive chemical raises cholesterol levels.
> Carbon Monoxide – this potentially poisonous gas reduces the levels of oxygen in the body.

Smoking can reduce your life expectancy dramatically - by as much as seven to eight years.

Some of the illnesses known to be contributed to by smoking, include:

Vascular disease

Smoking is one of the causes of this disease which is where the arteries harden progressively. This can lead to blood clots, which if they occur in the heart or brain, can be fatal. Forms of the disease include:

Coronary Thrombosis

This is when a blood clot occurs in the arteries which lead to the heart. This can cause a heart attack which can be fatal.

Cerebral Thrombosis

This is where the blood vessels leading to the brain become blocked which can cause a stroke, paralysis or collapse.

Other complications of the condition include kidney failure, high blood pressure and gangrene – which can lead to amputation.

Cancer

Ninety percent of lung cancers are caused by smoking. Throat cancer and mouth cancer are also common in smokers. The risk of cancer increases with the number of cigarettes you smoke in a day, how long you have smoked for, and how deeply you inhale.

Chronic Obstructive Pulmonary Disease

Also referred to as COPD, this is a group of conditions which impair the breathing such as emphysema and bronchitis.

Some of the other risks of smoking are:

High blood pressure.
Fertility problems.
Worsening of asthma.
Bloodshot and itchy eyes.
Macular degeneration.
Cataracts.
Stained teeth and gums.
Periodontal disease.
Ulcers.
Erectile dysfunction.

Passive smoking

It is not just the smoker who is affected by the negative impact of cigarettes. Passive smoking can affect others, particularly children who live in the same house as one or more adults who smoke. They run the risk of a higher chance of having asthma or bronchitis. Passive smoking also increases the risk of cot death.

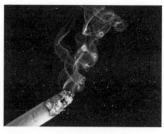

Giving up

If you take the decision to give up smoking it is reassuring to know that there are lots of resources available to help you. By going to visit your GP, you may be able to get nicotine patches on prescription or maybe even other medication to help you wean yourself off cigarettes. Some of the benefits of giving up are:

> Saving money – if you smoke 20 a day, this is equal to more than £2,500 a year.
>
> Better sex – your blood flow improves which increases sensitivity.
>
> Improved fertility – non smokers find it easier to become pregnant.
>
> Younger looking skin – without cigarettes your skin will receive more nutrients and facial ageing will be slowed.
>
> Whiter teeth – smoking stains your teeth.
>
> Better breathing – you won't get so out of breath going up the stairs.
>
> Longer life – stopping smoking adds years to your life expectancy.
>
> Less stress – nicotine addiction increases stress levels.
>
> Improved senses – your sense of smell and taste will recover.
>
> More energy – your circulation will improve and there will be more oxygen in your system.

Things that will help you give up include signing up to the NHS Stop Smoking Service and alternative therapies can be very helpful, particularly hypnotherapy and acupuncture which have helped many others achieve successful results.

Staying healthy during a hospital stay

Take proactive steps to prevent infections such as MRSA and C. difficile. Wash your hands regularly and use the gel sprays and hand gels that are readily available in hospitals. Make sure your visitors do this as well. Ask your visitors not to come into the hospital if they are ill. Limit the number of visitors that you have.

Follow ward advice regarding food, flowers and laundry. It is usually a good idea to take dirty clothes home with you in a sealed plastic bag and wash them using a cycle of at least 60 degrees. You should also wash any cuddly toys.

Don't fiddle around with dressings, catheters or drips. Take a new pair of slippers into hospital with you. Don't walk around in bare feet. Keep your area around your part of the ward tidy.

If you know that you have a stay in hospital coming up then make sure you eat especially healthily in the run-up to your admission. This will help boost your immune system and ensure that you are in the best shape for any treatment.

Tell staff about past and present infections and any antibiotics you are taking.

By following all of these guidelines whilst you are in hospital then you can ensure that you have the best chance of staying healthy, being strong enough to ensure that your treatment is successful and minimising your chances of having to go to hospital again in the future.

Within each of us lies the power of our consent to health and sickness, to riches and poverty, to freedom and to slavery. It is we who control these, and not another.

Richard Boch

Thirteen:
Make Health Your Priority

Have regular check-ups, medical examinations and blood tests

Most people only visit their doctor when they have a problem. Some people only take their car to the mechanic when the car has developed a problem. However most people have their cars serviced regularly and therefore the car mechanic can spot problems in advance or early enough to prevent a major problem happening at all.

When the car is 3 years old, it has to have a yearly MOT, which is a thorough check of all the main car parts. Would it not make more sense if we have our bodies checked out at regular intervals and say a yearly bodily MOT? If we have a six monthly or yearly full medical examination, blood and urine tests, the chances are, if our bodies were not completely healthy, then medical problems would be picked up at an early stage and in the majority of cases our medical problems could be cured or controlled.

If you are feeling unwell, get good medical advice as early as possible

If you are feeling unwell and you believe it is more than a minor ailment, like a cold or flu, then prepare and write down your symptoms and any other relevant information and make an appointment to see your doctor.

Make sure that during your appointment with your doctor that they give you the time you need to have your say and that the doctor is allowing time to make a proper diagnosis. When they give you their opinion as to what may be the problem and treatment, if any, ask them questions so that you understand fully the diagnosis and treatment.

Before having a medical procedure, make sure that the doctor explains it fully to you. If you are elderly, nervous, or indeed you would just be happier taking a friend or relative with you to your appointment, then do so. It makes sense to have an extra mouth, an extra set of ears and an extra pair of eyes. Your friend can also ask questions of the doctor and remember important information that you may have forgotten.

Be an educated patient

If you do become a patient, make sure that you are an educated patient. You need to have a good understanding about your illness and your treatment. That way you can ask relevant and important questions, you will understand what is being said and explained to you and you will be aware of other treatment options.

Be aware that doctors do not always get it right. They are not infallible and they can be guilty of not giving their patients the time and attention they deserve; so take more of a major role in your own health issues, know your rights and do not hesitate if you need to be more assertive.

Funding for the Health Service

With the economies of the United Kingdom and Ireland being in such a state, funding for health care will no doubt be considerably reduced and there will be little new investment for health care, to help it keep pace

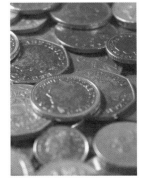

with new developments, new treatments and highly qualified staff.

We can be pretty certain that health care will suffer and the users of the Health Service will suffer also. With the pressure on finances, there will be staff cutbacks, cancelled operations, longer waiting lists, ward closures and restrictions on the prescribing of new drug treatments.

' :: in turn will cause low morale and caring standards will fall. It is now essential that in order to get quality health treatment and care you will need to be better informed, more vigilant and become an educated patient.

Ask for your test results

When you have medical tests carried out, including blood and urine tests, enquire when the results will be available. When the results arrive, ring your doctor's surgery and ask for the findings. Make a note of things like cholesterol levels and other readings so that you can compare them with your next results.

If any of the results are outside of the normal range, see your doctor and ask for a full explanation and what treatment, if any, you need to commence. Make sure that you fully understand the abnormal test results, the implications of them and any treatment that is necessary.

Try and anticipate what to expect from tests, operations, procedures and treatments in advance. You can do most of the research on the Internet and the more you know in advance, the more likely you will be to notice if something isn't right.

If you do not understand something then ask for a full explanation and ask as many questions as it takes. The more you know and understand the greater empowered you will be and the respect your doctor has for you will rise.

Read the literature on any medication you are taking

Any medication that you are prescribed by your doctor will come with an information leaflet, which gives you all the details you need to know about the medication.

Make sure you read this and pay particular attention to the side effects and the contraindications. The side effects will alert you to any dangers the medication may have. If you experience any of these side effects, inform your doctor who will take any action necessary.

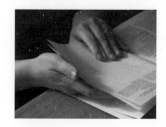

The contraindications will tell you when this medication should not be taken, e.g. during pregnancy, if you have a certain medical condition or if you are already taking another medication with which it may react badly. On most occasions your doctor should pick this up, but just in case they don't, make it your responsibility to read the literature.

Be polite but assertive with your doctor

When you make a visit to your doctor all too often you will leave feeling that you have been rushed and/or that you have been given very little chance to contribute to the conversation. Doctors work very busy schedules and they may be under pressure to make up lost time.

This being the case you may only have been given a few minutes in order to have a diagnosis made and treatment decided. You may find that you leave your doctor's surgery more anxious than when you arrived. So, always be polite but assertive with your doctor. Every day patients are visiting their doctors with what might be the start of a life-threatening illness and time constraints may contribute to a wrong diagnosis being made.

Do all that you can to see that this doesn't happen and if you are not happy, make a further appointment to see your doctor, or arrange to have a second opinion. Sometimes when we are in the company of a doctor, or in hospital, we can feel helpless, as if we are completely in their care and under their control.

They have a power over you. Also some doctors can be quite arrogant and make you feel hesitant about speaking, feeling that you should just sit there and be quiet, feeling vulnerable. Don't let this happen to you.

Don't be afraid to ask for a second opinion

If you are not happy with your doctor, for whatever reason, tell them that you want a second opinion. You may feel that your doctor has not diagnosed you properly, is working outside their level of competence, is a junior doctor who lacks experience, is not taking you seriously, is not listening to you, or is not giving you adequate time.

Perhaps you just don't like their attitude. No matter what your reason is, feel free to ask for a second opinion. You are entitled to do so and this should not be a problem for your doctor. Medical errors and misdiagnosis are more likely to happen when the doctor is inexperienced, fatigued, has time pressures, is stressed or is overworked.

Find a top consultant who specialises in your medical problem

If you have an ongoing medical problem or an illness that you believe may not be diagnosed correctly, it is in your interest to find out who the top consultants are, who specialise in your particular medical problem and which hospitals they work in.

It may be a good idea to get your general practitioner to refer you to them, or you can seek a private consultation with them directly. If you are anxious about your medical condition, or you feel that your doctor is spending very little time with you, or the treatment you are getting doesn't seem to be making any difference, then make an appointment to see the best consultant that you can find.

Even if you have to pay for the initial consultation, it will be money well spent. There are many excellent doctors working in the Health Service and in the private sector and with the use of the Internet they are not too difficult to find.

Whatever your medical condition, become an expert

No matter what your medical condition is, within a short period of time you can carry out research on the Internet or in your local library and end up knowing as much, if not more, about your medical condition than your own doctor does.

You will certainly have more passion and time to research all about your condition and treatment than your doctor does. Although there is a wealth of medical knowledge on the Internet, I am not suggesting that you make your doctor redundant, or that you try and diagnose or treat yourself.

However you can carry out enough research that will help you understand any medical condition that you have and the possible treatments. It will also give you an indication if your doctor's diagnosis makes sense.

Research the treatments that are available for your medical condition

Carry out regular research in order to find out what treatments are available throughout the world, and what new treatments there are in the pipeline. There could be more successful treatments for your medical condition than you are receiving from your doctor.

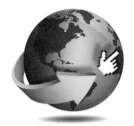

Your doctor may be strongly influenced by the cost of the treatment and working within the constraints of a budget and you may be receiving the lower cost treatment, and not necessarily the best treatment. Therefore don't assume that the treatment your doctor has prescribed is the best that money can buy.

Make it your responsibility to find the best treatment available for you or a family member, and then set about getting it.

Request that your general practitioner sends you to the best specialist available

Thousands of patients have suffered with medical conditions for years that have caused them pain, discomfort and embarrassment yet, despite repeated visits to their doctor, nothing seems to be done.

Their doctor continues with treatments that do little or nothing for the patient and they don't bother to send their patients to specialists who will help them. Sometimes you wonder if some family doctors realise that the specialists exist.

There is a television programme called Embarrassing Bodies, where people come to a mobile unit which is staffed by doctors and travels around the UK. They call it Embarrassing Bodies because people, with a wide range of unusual and longstanding medical problems, present themselves to these doctors for help.

It makes me wonder what these peoples' general practitioners have been doing for them over the years. In most cases, it would seem to be very little. Yet these mobile doctors, in most of the cases, get them the help they need to cure their medical problem or to make it considerably better.

We can only conclude that there are a considerable number of general practitioners who are too busy to get their patients the help and treatment they so desperately need. In 2001 the then President of the General Medical Council described the medical profession as a 'secretive and paternalistic culture' with a 'lack of respect' for patients.

Look after yourself – alcohol, tobacco, diet and exercise

It would be wrong to leave all the responsibility for staying healthy to the Health Service. We have to take responsibility for our own health and actions and avoid doing anything that may damage our bodies.

We know, without doubt, that tobacco products can damage us in many different ways. Excessive consumption of alcohol could lead us to become addicted and can seriously affect our physical and mental health. Keeping ourselves healthy is not only about avoiding alcohol, tobacco, fats etc., it is also about doing things.

Eating a well-balanced healthy diet, keeping our weight within normal limits and dealing with stress helps to contribute to a good lifestyle. As well, regular exercise is essential and can play a major role in maintaining our health.

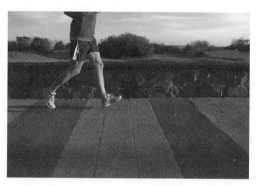

Life's priorities – health, relationships, career and money.

The priorities in most people's lives are to have a great job or career, earn enough money to pay all the debts, have a wonderful lifestyle and a rewarding and loving relationship with their family.

However, it would seem that the majority of people take their health for granted and don't have it as a major priority in their lives. If you don't have your health, then the other priorities can become meaningless. Our health and well-being are so important that we have to make a conscious effort to strive to do all we can to maintain our good health.

Start putting your health at the top of your priority list. You won't regret it.

A positive mental attitude

Most of us have heard stories about the power of the mind, mind over matter and the law of attraction (we attract what we think about). It is fair to say that a positive mental attitude can make a difference.

When it comes to your health and other parts of your life, always try to be positive, be a fighter and never give in. With a positive mental attitude you may be surprised as to what you can achieve. In all aspects of your life it always helps if you keep company with positive people.

Remember - doctors and nurses are only human

Like all humans they make mistakes. But unlike most humans, some of the mistakes that doctors and nurses make can prove to be very costly, not for themselves, but for you the patient.

Do not take their skills for granted and minimise the effect of their mistakes on your life. All doctors and nurses make mistakes and, though it is reasonable to assume that the more qualified, skilled and experienced the doctor or nurse is, the less mistakes they'll make. However even they make costly mistakes.

Just look out for your health and be alert and mindful when in any healthcare setting. If mistakes are made they could change your life or even worse.

Some causes of medical errors and misdiagnosis

Inexperienced doctors.

Delayed diagnosis.

Poor communication between doctor, nurse and patient (one party may not be fluent in English).

Lack of communication between GP, consultant, nurse, laboratory, etc..

Doctors or nurses suffering from sleep deprivation.

New or experimental treatments or procedures.

Illegible handwriting.

Performing the wrong surgery.

Incorrect prescriptions.

Taking more than one drug that will interact dangerously with each other.

Inadequate assessment of the patient.

Prescribing drugs with names that sound or look alike.

Apart from the cases that are reported by the media, doctors regularly make mistakes and their colleagues who may be aware of them, because of the nature of the medical profession, rarely report them. More needs to be done by the medical and nursing professions to greatly reduce the numbers of medical errors and to introduce safeguards that will help prevent avoidable deaths and injuries.

Avoid being stressed

One of the major enemies of our health is stress. Stress can cause illness and disease and make any medical condition we have worse. It can make our lives hell and do the same to those people who are close to us.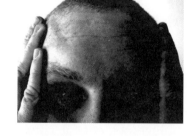

We all should have ways to deal with stress or to prevent ourselves from becoming stressed. It is good to have a relaxing hobby or pastime. Meditation, relaxation, yoga, walking and other similar activities and hobbies can be great stress busters and can help in preventing the onset of stress.

Ensure that you're treated with dignity and respect

Doctors, nurses and other healthcare workers are often guilty of treating their patients like a number or a piece of meat and forget that their patients are human beings by not showing them the respect that they would want and expect if they were in your shoes.

Remember it is your right to be treated with dignity and respect and never accept anything less. You are a human being and never let anyone forget that. This is especially true in relation to people who are elderly. We often read about elderly people being abused in this way in hospitals and nursing homes.

Be involved in decisions about your care and treatment

Don't be totally trusting when it comes to your life. Of course, there will be times when we need the services of nurses and medical staff, but always make sure you are an equal partner in your health care and not just a bystander.

Make sure that you are fully involved in decisions about and in the ongoing care and treatment of any healthcare problem you may have. Remember, you are the senior partner for it is your life that is on the line.

If you are unhappy with your treatment, complain

Don't accept substandard healthcare or treatment. Make sure that you are always treated with respect and that the care and treatment you receive is of the highest possible standard.

Some doctors make it difficult for you to ask questions about your state of health and treatment. Considering the limited time you have with your doctor and perhaps feeling that they are under pressure from other patients waiting to see them, it is difficult to establish a meaningful relationship and be relaxed enough to ask the questions you would like answers to.

It is a terrible feeling leaving your doctor's surgery knowing that you had many other questions you needed answers to. Sometimes it helps to take a family member or friend to the appointment with you.

Have a plan

Prior to your appointment with the doctor or other healthcare professional, have a plan in your mind so that you can give your input and ask a number of questions you need answers to regarding your diagnosis and treatment.

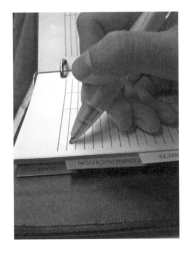

Be assertive and don't let anyone talk down to you or ignore what you are saying. If you wish, take a list of questions with you and have a pad and pen so that you can write down any important points that arise.

Don't be intimidated by your doctor

Some doctors can be quite arrogant and rude to their patients showing them little warmth or eye contact. This in itself only makes a patient more anxious and doesn't create a very therapeutic atmosphere. Some doctors can make it difficult for you to ask them questions about your state of health and treatment.

If this is the case with you, then you should discuss these difficulties with your doctor or else switch to a doctor who is more welcoming and friendly and who will allay your anxiety rather than heightening it.

What would you do, doctor?

If you need an appointment to see a specialist as well as doing your own research to find out who is the best specialist to see, ask your doctor if they had your medical complaint which specialist would they want to see. It can point you in the right direction.

Leave no stone unturned until you are diagnosed correctly

It is as much your responsibility as it is your doctor's to see that this happens. If your doctor refers you to a specialist, you should then take the initiative and if you haven't received an appointment with the specialist within two to three weeks, ring the specialist's secretary to enquire about your appointment.

If you are not getting an appointment soon tell them that you will take a cancellation, in order to get your appointment quicker. Ring the specialist's secretary every two weeks until you get your appointment.

If you are seeing a specialist or having tests carried out, make sure that it is given urgent attention and happens as quickly as possible.

This can't happen soon enough. If you are unable to have your initial appointment with the specialist, then consider paying for an initial appointment privately.

See a consultant, not a junior doctor

Not only getting an appointment at the earliest possible time is important, but seeing a consultant rather than a junior doctor is also of the utmost importance. Always strive to see the best possible doctor and get the best possible treatment.

Seeing the best qualified, most skilled, most experienced and most senior doctor should increase your odds for a more successful outcome.

Elderly, disabled and vulnerable patients

In most cases it is a good idea for people who are elderly, disabled or vulnerable to have a health advocate. This could be a family member, friend or a volunteer or someone who has some understanding and knowledge of the NHS, doctors, and how the system works. Also it is better if the advocate is observant and assertive. Get them to accompany you when visiting your doctor or outpatient's department, or if you are an inpatient in hospital.

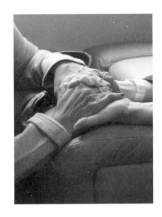

Cancer, heart disease, stroke and medical errors

When we take ill and need to have tests and investigations, the concern uppermost in our minds is the dread of having cancer, heart disease and other serious illnesses that may threaten our lives.

Few of us would consider another serious life-threatening scenario – medical errors and hospital blunders. Unfortunately, medical errors and hospital blunders cost thousands of people their lives every year and leave thousands chronically ill or injured. When receiving treatment from your doctor or hospital, always be vigilant and alert about the treatment you are having and the standard of care you are receiving.

Recurring symptoms

If you have recurring symptoms and they don't disappear, nor are they helped by initial treatments you have been given by your doctor, then ask for a second opinion and further investigations and insist on being seen by a top specialist. The sooner you are correctly diagnosed and start the proper treatment regimen the better.

Accurate diagnosis

Thousands of patients each year are incorrectly diagnosed. Many of these patients have life-threatening illnesses that may not be correctly diagnosed until some years later. No one can afford to be living with an illness that has not been properly diagnosed and is taking treatment that is not appropriate for the illness.

One of the worst things that can happen to a patient is to be incorrectly diagnosed, and then be diagnosed correctly when the illness is too advanced to be treated successfully. So always be proactive, take nothing for granted and leave nothing to chance.

Strive for an early diagnosis

It is of the utmost importance, when you are ill, that you should strive for an early diagnosis. An early diagnosis could save your life. Many diseases can be cured or stopped in their tracks if they are accurately diagnosed at an early stage. Each year thousands of patients, because of an incorrect early diagnosis, often receive treatment for years for a medical condition they do not have.

Some years later, having received the wrong treatment for the wrong illness, it comes to light that the patient has a more serious or terminal illness that is now untreatable. A correct early diagnosis of the illness when the symptoms first appear means there is a greater chance that the illness can be treated successfully. You probably know of someone within your family or circle of friends that this has happened to.

Time is of the essence

As the average general practitioner consultation lasts around seven minutes, you need to be prepared to make the best use of this short period of time. Prior to your appointment, keep a diary of all your symptoms, recurring problems, the side effects of any medication you are taking and any questions you want answered.

Bring your note pad with a list of all the above points to your appointment. It would be difficult to believe, considering that consultations with family doctors last an average of seven minutes, how a doctor could possibly always be accurate with the diagnosis and treatment. It helps us to understand why the first diagnosis is not always a correct diagnosis.

Make provision for good health care

We make many plans for our lives, yet somehow provision for health care takes a back seat. If a health problem arises, we are all at sea, lost and vulnerable. Maybe it's time to rethink, to refocus and to reprioritise. Our health is one of the most important things in our lives and should always come first.

Health is my expected Heaven.

John Keats

Fourteen: Conclusions

As we have examined during the course of this book, doctors and other healthcare staff undergo extensive training which is ongoing throughout their professional lives.

They are regulated by professional bodies and are subject to the same laws as you or I; as well as by professional codes of conduct.

Whilst most of the time doctors and nurses do a wonderful job of helping us with our medical problems, not all healthcare staff are good at their job. Just like the rest of us they sometimes have bad days, they become ill or have things on their mind. We have already seen that staff and equipment shortages can cause issues for patients.

We have looked at how hospitals are run, the departments that they are made up of and the staff that you may encounter during your stay. We have also seen how food, parking and security can all have an impact on you during your time in hospital. The impact of hospital infections has been set out with details from the high profile case of Leslie Ash.

Drugs and the pharmaceutical industry were examined, and the way that the drug companies work closely with doctors was laid out. Different types of medication and their side effects were detailed. The role of pharmacists was explained and the services that you can find in your local pharmacy were highlighted.

The structure of the NHS was explained, with the differences between primary and secondary care identified. The private medical sector was also looked at, with common features of Private Medical Insurance and an explanation of how the process works.

Some of the incidents of medical failures that have occurred during the last few years were described, not as a way of scare-mongering, but as a way of raising awareness of what can go wrong.

We also looked at techniques that you can use to be assertive with the medical and nursing staff who are dealing with you. Assertiveness is an important skill when dealing with doctors because it helps you to be on the same level as them. We looked at how you can research and gain knowledge so you can take ownership of your own health and make sure that you are in charge of what happens to your body.

Living a healthy lifestyle was where we looked at how we can take care of ourselves in the best possible way to ensure that we minimise our chances of getting serious illnesses. Nutrition, exercise and healthy habits were looked at in detail with plenty of suggestions on how to incorporate health into your day to day lifestyle.

Make your health your priority was our final chapter, where we asked you to rethink the importance that you give to your health, to understand it more and to become a champion of your own health care.

In summary, we can conclude that we have an excellent healthcare system available to us here in the UK. It is, on the whole, staffed by responsible and professional people. We must, however, retain control over what is happening to us and not just blindly lie back and let the medical profession treat us without our full involvement.

The greatest wealth is health.

Virgil

Medical Qualifications

BC, BCh Bachelor of Surgery
BChir Bachelor of Surgery
BDA British Dental Association
BM Bachelor of Medicine
BMedSci Bachelor of Medical Sciences
BPharm Bachelor of Pharmacy
BS Bachelor of Surgery
ChB Bachelor of Surgery
CPH Certificate in Public Health
DA Diploma in Anaesthetics
DAvMed Diploma in Aviation Medicine
DCh Doctor of Surgery
DCH Diploma in Child Health
DCP Diploma in Clinical Pathology
DCPath Diploma of the College of Pathologists
DDS Doctor of Dental Surgery
DFHom Diploma of the Faculty of Homoeopathy
DFM Diploma in Forensic Medicine
DGM Diploma in Geriatric Medicine
DGO Diploma in Gynaecology and Obstetrics
Dip GU Med Diploma in Genitourinary Medicine
DMR Diploma in Medical Radiology
DO Diploma in Ophthalmology
DObst Diploma in Obstetrics
DPath Diploma in Pathology
DPhysMed Diploma in Physical Medicine
DPH Diploma in Public Health
DPM Diploma in Psychological Medicine
DR Diploma in Radiology
DRACOG Diploma of the Royal Australian College of Obstetricians and Gynaecologists
DRACR Diploma of the Royal Australasian College of Radiologists
DRCOG Diploma of the Royal College of Obstetricians and Gynaecologists
DRCPath Diploma of the Royal College of Pathologists
DS Doctor of Surgery
F1 Foundation Year 1
F2 Foundation Year 2
FFA Fellow of the Faculty of Anaesthetists
FFCM Fellow of the Faculty of Community Medicine
FFFP Fellow of the Faculty of Family Planning

FFHom Fellow of the Faculty of Homoeopathy
FFPath Fellow of the Faculty of Pathology
FFPHM Fellow of the Faculty of Public Health Medicine
FFR Fellow of the Faculty of Radiologists
FRACGP Fellow of the Royal Australian College of General Practitioners
FRACO Fellow of the Royal Australasian College of Ophthalmologists
FRACOG Fellow of the Royal Australian College of Obstetricians and Gynaecologists
FRACP Fellow of the Royal Australasian College of Physicians
FRACR Fellow of the Royal Australasian College of Radiologists
FRACS Fellow of the Royal Australasian College of Surgeons
FRANZCP Fellow of the Royal Australian and New Zealand College of Psychiatrists
FRCA Fellow of the Royal College of Anaesthetists
FRCGP Fellow of the Royal College of General Practitioners
FRCOG Fellow of the Royal College of Obstetricians and Gynaecologists
FRCOphth Fellow of the College of Ophthalmology
FRCPA Fellow of the Royal College of Pathologists of Australia
FRCPath Fellow of the Royal College of Pathologists
FRCPI Fellow of the Royal College of Physicians of Ireland
FRCPS Fellow of the Royal College of Physicians & Surgeons
FRCPsych Fellow of the Royal College of Psychiatrists
FRCR Fellow of the Royal College of Radiologists
FRCS Fellow of the Royal College of Surgeons
FRCSI Fellow of the Royal College of Surgeons of Ireland
FRS Fellow of the Royal Society
FRSH Fellow of the Royal Society of Health
GP General Practitioner
Honorary e.g. Honorary Consultant Cardiologist – Consultant with academic/ research responsibilities
LCPS Licentiate of the College of Physicians & Surgeons
LMS Licentiate of Medicine & Surgery
LMSSA Licentiate in Medicine & Surgery – Society of Apothecaries London
LRCP Licentiate of the Royal College of Physicians
LRCPI Licentiate of the Royal College of Physicians of Ireland
LRCPS Licentiate of the Royal College of Physicians & Surgeons
LRCS Licentiate of the Royal College of Surgeons
LRCSI Licentiate of the Royal College of Surgeons of Ireland
LSA Licentiate of the Society of Apothecaries London
MACGP Member of the Australasian College of General Practitioners
MACO Member of the Australian College of Ophthalmologists
MBA Master of Business Administration

MBAcA Member of the British Acupuncture Association
MBBCh Bachelor of Medicine and Bachelor of Surgery
MBBS Bachelor of Medicine and Bachelor of Surgery
MBChB Bachelor of Medicine and Bachelor of Surgery
MCh Master of Surgery
MChir Master of Surgery
MChOrth Master of Orthopaedic Surgery
MClinPscychol Master of Clinical Psychology
MD Doctor of Medicine
MFFP Member of the Faculty of Family Planning
MFHom Member of the Faculty of Homoeopathy
MFOM Member of the Faculty of Occupational Medicine
MFPHM Member of the Faculty of Public Health Medicine
MMed Master of Medicine
MMedSc Master of Medical Science
MRACP Member of the Royal Australasian College of Physicians
MRCGP Member of the Royal College of General Practitioners
MRCOG Member of the Royal College of Obstetricians and Gynaecologists
MRCP Member of the Royal College of Physicians
MRCPath Member of the Royal College of Pathologists
MRCPI Member of the Royal College of Physicians of Ireland
MRCPsych Member of the Royal College of Psychiatrists
MRCS Member of the Royal College of Surgeons
MRNZCGP Member of the Royal New Zealand College of General Practitioners
MS Master of Surgery
PRHO Pre-Registration House Officer (now replaced by Foundation Year 1)
SAS Staff and Associate Specialist
StR Specialty Registrar

(Source: British Medical Association, 2008)

Age does not depend upon years, but upon temperament and health. Some men are born old and some never grow so.

Tryon Edwards

Bibliography

Association of British Insurers
*www.abi.org.uk/Information/Consumers/Health_and_Protection/Useful_downloads_
Health_and_Protection_Insurance.aspx*

BBC, 'Tweeting' medics expose patients
news.bbc.co.uk/1/hi/8266546.stm

BBC, Medical records found in corridor
news.bbc.co.uk/1/hi/scotland/glasgow_and_west/7978368.stm

BBC, Doctors Need More Drugs Training
news.bbc.co.uk/1/hi/health/7844397.stm

Bennett, R., Health News: Times Online
www.timesonline.co.uk/tol/news/uk/health/article5965535.ece

British Heart Foundation, What is a Healthy Diet?
*www.bhf.org.uk/Keeping_your_heart_healthy/healthy_eating/what_is_a_healthy_diet.
aspx*

British Medical Association, Doctors Training and Qualifications
www.bma.org.uk/patients_public/doctorsqual.jsp

BUPA, Improving Assertiveness
hcd2.bupa.co.uk/fact_sheets/html/improving_assertiveness.html

Carvel, J., Learning Disability
www.guardian.co.uk/society/2009/mar/24/neglect-nhs-learning-disabilities

Department of Health, Committee of Enquiry to investigate how the NHS
handled allegations about the performance and conduct of Richard Neale,
London, 2004

Edwards, T., Sharing patient records would be 'ethical but illegal'
*www.thefirstpost.co.uk/48388,news-comment,news-politics,doctors-ditch-patient-
confidentiality-research-gmc-ethics-illegal-eu-law-nhs-privacy-data-protection*

Gordan, S., An Overview of The Pharmaceutical Industry in the UK
www.allaboutmedicalsales.com/articles/pharma_overview_jt_250102.html

Henderson, R., A to Z of Hospital Departments
netdoctor.co.uk/health-services-guide/hospital-departments.htm

Mencap briefing on Martin Ryan
www.mencap.org.uk/document.asp?id=9610

NHS Careers, Training To Become A Doctor
www.nhscareers.nhs.uk/details/Default.aspx?Id=561

NHS Core Principles
www.nhs.uk/NHSEngland/aboutnhs/Pages/NHSCorePrinciples.aspx

NHS Structure
www.nhs.uk/nhsengland/aboutnhs/pages/NHSstructure.aspx

Ormondroyd, Jan, Achieving Age Equality in Health and Social Care, a report to the Secretary of State for Health, October 2009

Parliamentary and Health Service Ombudsman, Six lives: the provision of public services to people with learning disabilities, London 2009

Paul, M. W., Healthy Eating, Tips for a healthy diet and better nutrition
helpguide.org/life/healthy_eating_diet.htm

Private Healthcare UK, Medical Training of UK doctors and specialists
www.privatehealth.co.uk/privatespecialists/medical-training/

Rosenthal, M., *The Incompetent Doctor*, Open University Press, 1995
Smith, M., *When I Say No I Feel Guilty*, 1975

The Daily Telegraph, Health News
www.telegraph.co.uk/health/healthnews/6318299/Couple-receive-160000-over-hospitals-baby-blunders.html

The Sunday Times, Health
www.timesonline.co.uk/tol/life_and_style/health/article6869646.ece

Money is the most envied but the least enjoyed. Health is the most enjoyed but the least envied.

Charles Caleb Cotton